Nuclear Cardiology:
Selected Computer Aspects

Symposium Proceedings
Atlanta, Georgia, January 22–23, 1978
●
Sponsored by the Computer Council of
The Society of Nuclear Medicine

BOOK COORDINATOR

James A. Sorenson, Ph.D.
University of Utah Medical Center, Salt Lake City, Utah

SCIENTIFIC PROGRAM COMMITTEE

Stephen L. Bacharach, Ph.D., Chairman
National Institutes of Health, Bethesda, Maryland

Nathaniel M. Alpert, Ph.D.
Massachusetts General Hospital, Boston, Massachusetts

David M. Shames, M.D.
University of California, San Francisco, California

Published by THE SOCIETY OF NUCLEAR MEDICINE, INC.
475 Park Avenue South, New York, NY 10016

ISBN 0-932004-00-8

Library of Congress Number 78-58477.
Printed in the United States of America.

FOREWORD

Nuclear cardiology is a field of growing importance in nuclear medicine. This volume contains the proceedings of a symposium on nuclear cardiology, sponsored by the Computer Council of the Society of Nuclear Medicine, and held at Atlanta, Georgia, January 22-23, 1978. It presents up-to-date discussions of a variety of topics in nuclear cardiology. It is hoped that this publication will provide useful information on the present status of this rapidly-developing field.

Special thanks are due to Dr. Stephen Bacharach, program chairman for the symposium, and to the authors, for their efforts toward making the symposium a success and this publication possible; to Mr. Jim Swan, Ms. Micki Collins, and others at the central office of the Society of Nuclear Medicine for their help in the publication of this volume; and to Mrs. Janie Thomas for her patient secretarial assistance in editing and preparing the manuscripts for publication.

James A. Sorenson
Book Coordinator
Society of Nuclear Medicine

SELECTED COMPUTER ASPECTS OF NUCLEAR CARDIOLOGY:

AN INTRODUCTION TO THE PROCEEDINGS

Stephen L. Bacharach

National Institutes of Health
Bethesda, Maryland 20014

Many people have considered computers in nuclear medicine a solution in search of a problem. Nuclear medicine departments have often considered the advantages of a computer insufficient to justify its purchase. Within the last year or so, the sought after problem has been found. Nuclear cardiology has given us a clinically important problem which, very nearly, is ideally suited to our patiently waiting solution. For the first time there is a use for computers which is of sufficient clinical importance that the purchase of a minicomputer could probably be justified for that single use alone.

The great current interest in nuclear cardiology (in particular, gated equilibrium and first-pass techniques) is probably in large part due to the advantages of being able to obtain cardiac "movies," and calculate ejection fractions, quickly and non-invasively. The ability to observe (and quantitate) such data quickly has allowed the technique to be applied to intervention studies -- comparative studies performed during rest and exercise, or with and without drug administration. These studies, especially rest/exercise comparisons, have been shown to be diagnostically sensitive in the detection of ischemic coronary artery disease. In addition, there is evidence to indicate that the test may have important applications in the evaluation of therapy and in prognosis in several classes of cardiac disease.

The performance and interpretation of gated equilibrium and first-pass studies requires an understanding of the basic physical assumptions upon which the techniques are based. Additionally, such studies often put special demands on the instrumentation and computer software. One of the goals of this symposium was to examine the validity of these assumptions, to discuss the limitations of the current methodology, and to speculate on new instrumentation techniques.

The papers in the symposium fell into roughly three categories. The primary emphasis of the meeting was on gated equilibrium and first-pass techniques, and these papers comprised the majority of those presented. In addition, there were two briefer sessions, one concerning thallium-201 image processing and display, and the other dealing with shunt detection, modeling, and special techniques. Unfortunately, the proceedings contain only the papers, and not the discussions which followed them.

The first four papers should give the reader an overview of the clinical possibilities of both first pass and gated equilibrium studies: Intervention studies -- rest/exercise; drug intervention; pre-op/post-op comparisons; right ventricular function assessment; wall motion studies. The fifth paper compares the imaging techniques used in the above papers to similar measurements made without a gamma camera. These non-imaging, or "temporal imaging" methods, in addition to being of great interest and potential in their own right, serve to illustrate some of the problems and limitations of both imaging and non-imaging techniques. The next group of papers (6-11) addresses these potential difficulties. How can background be adequately adjusted for? Is counting rate truly proportional to volume? What are the effects of beat length fluctuations? What timing resolution is required for a clinically accurate volume curve? How critical is region of interest selection? Finally, the last three papers of the first session (12-14) dis-

cuss the feasibility of eliminating the most time-consuming portion of data analysis -- manually selecting the ventricular and background region of interest. If the computer could be made to reliably perform this task, a nearly totally automated study would be possible, perhaps significantly reducing the variability intrinsic to subjective visual determinations.

The first of the two briefer sessions (papers 15-16) deals with the ability of the computer to enhance the clinical utility of T1-201 studies by cine-graphic display techniques, and image processing. The final session contains a description of a methodology for automated shunt detection by the method of gamma variates (paper 19), as well as two somewhat unusual and interesting applications to nuclear cardiology (papers 17 and 18). In the first of these (paper 17) a novel form of analysis is described which allows calculations of ejection fraction from a low temporal resolution first pass study. In the second paper (#18), a model is developed which may allow region of interest curves to be corrected for extraneous counts arising from scatter and chamber overlap. Finally, the last paper (#20), discusses a display system optimized for nuclear cardiology.

It is usually unwise to draw definitive conclusions in a field as rapidly evolving as nuclear cardiology. Tomorrow's data may well alter today's conclusions. In addition, different people may well arrive at somewhat different conclusions after having listened to the same presentations. With the above facts in mind, the following represents one observer's view of the conclusions that might be drawn from the presented papers and discussions. Included are only those points about which some concensus seemed to have been reached. It is by no means complete and is limited to the first portion of the program.

Clinical data from both first-transit and gated equilibrium techniques were presented. Both techniques seem to give very similar quantitative results for rest/exercise left ventricular function (LV) studies, when ejection fraction is used as the comparator. First-pass techniques may additionally be able to evaluate right ventricular function, while equilibrium studies seem best suited for multiple intervention studies.

Very high count rates are necessary for adequate first-transit studies. The dead times from single crystal cameras would seem, at first, to preclude such studies with conventional Anger cameras. Data was presented, however, which indicated that this may not be the case. Conventional single crystal cameras, although sustaining significant count losses, may well respond quite adequately under the usual conditions of a first-transit measurement.

Ejection fraction and qualitative wall motion evaluation from cinematic display seem to be the primary use to which first-pass and gated equilibrium studies are put. If ejection fraction is the only quantitative information of interest, it appears that a framing rate of approximately 25-30 frames per cardiac cycle is sufficient. Other quantities (ejection and filling rates, timing parameters, etc.) derived from the LV activity curve may also prove to be of clinical utility. To accurately determine these quantities, higher framing rates may prove necessary.

Data was presented which indicated that counting rate may not be precisely proportional to ventricular volume, due primarily to self attenuation effects. Such effects may produce small but measurable systematic errors in count based ejection fractions calculated from first-transit or gated equilibrium studies.

Fluctuations in heart rate in a patient in sinus rhythm were shown to produce no significant variations in any of the previously mentioned quantities derivable from the LV time activity curve. The exception to this is with patients in atrial fibrillation. In such patients, even when a beat (or beats) of a single length are used, it is unclear as to whether these particular beats truly characterize the patient.

The largest source of random error in the determination of the LV ejection fraction seems due to variations in defining the background region of interest. In general it seems more important to use a reproducible method of background determination than to strive for one which is absolutely correct but subject to large inter-observer variations. To a lesser extent, fluctuations in the location of the LV region of interest may also produce errors. Computer generated regions of interest seem to produce excellent agreement with manually drawn areas in most patients. Such automated techniques do not, of course, possess "interobserver" fluctuations. In a significant number of patients, however, the computer may be capable of isolating the LV. Thus, human observation of the computer's area is still a necessary component of most semi-automated systems. Evidence was also presented that indicated multiple LV regions of interest, whose size varies over the cardiac cycle, may produce higher (and possibly more accurate) ejection fractions, in first-transit measurements. It is possible similar conclusions may hold for equilibrium studies.

Nuclear cardiology has brought renewed interest to the use of computers in nuclear medicine. At present, the ability to perform first-pass and gated equilibrium studies is available primarily as part of a much more elaborate nuclear medicine computer system. Relatively recent technological improvements, such as low cost, high density computer memory, may cause this situation to change, considerably expanding the use of nuclear cardiology procedures in the future.

NUCLEAR CARDIOLOGY:

SELECTED COMPUTER ASPECTS

CONTENTS   PAGE

CONTENTS   PAGE

COMPUTER-BASED RADIONUCLIDE CINEANGIOGRAPHY DURING EXERCISE[*]

Jeffrey S. Borer, M.D.[†], Stephen L. Bacharach, Ph.D.,
Michael V. Green, M.S., Kenneth M. Kent, M.D., Ph.D.,
Stephen E. Epstein, M.D., Gerald S. Johnston, M.D.

From the Cardiology Branch, National Heart, Lung, and Blood Institute,
and the Department of Nuclear Medicine, Clinical Center
National Institutes of Health, Bethesda, Maryland.

ABSTRACT

   Our previously reported real-time, computer-based system for creation of
$99m$Tc ECG-gated cardiac cineangiograms permits acquisition of visually interpretable movies (for regional left ventricular function (RLVF) analysis) and
statistically reliable high temporal resolution time-activity curves (for LV
ejection fraction (EF) analysis) during 1-2 minutes of intense exercise. In
normal subjects, EF invariably increases during exercise, and no RLVF abnormalities occur. In contrast, in patients with coronary artery disease
exercise almost invariably induces RLVF abnormalities, and reductions in EF,
even in asymptomatic patients; both nitroglycerin and coronary artery bypass
grafting can improve EF and RLVF during exericse. In patients with aortic
regurgitation, exercise induces abnormalities in EF not only in symptomatic
patients, but in many asymptomatic patients as well, a finding which may aid
in appropriate timing of therapy in the latter group. Thus radionuclide
cineangiography is of major clinical utility in the functional assessment of
patients with cardiac disease.

---

[*] Presented as "Evaluation of clinical utility of real-time computer-based
   radionuclide cineangiography" at Computers in Cardiology, 1977, sponsored
   by IEEE Computer Society, and reprinted, with permission, from proceedings
   of IEEE Computer Society, 1977. (In press)
[†] Address for reprints: Jeffrey S. Borer, M.D., National Institutes of Health,
   Bldg. 10, Room 7B-15, Bethesda, MD. 20014

INTRODUCTION

Recently we have reported a computed based system for the creation of ECG-gated cardiac cineangiograms (1-4) modified to permit simultaneous acquisition and display of data in real time (5-6). The system permits acquisition of 20,000 events per second. Hence, in one to two minutes information is acquired that provides visually interpretable movies, suitable for analysis of regional left ventricular function, and statistically reliable time activity curves with high (10-msec) temporal resolution, suitable for precise assessment of global ejection fraction.

With minor modifications, this system has been adapted for use during exercise (7-14). Clinically, this represents a potentially important development, since in patients with heart disease, even when anatomical abnormalities are relatively severe, left ventricular function often is normal or near normal with the patient at rest. Commonly, left ventricular functional reserve is exceeded only during stress, such as that imposed by exercise, and it is only in this situation that the functional severity of any cardiac disease can be accurately assessed.

Since developing the exercise technique two years age, we have performed clinical trials in over 600 patients with various forms of heart disease (7-14). These studies have demonstrated the practical clinical utility of radionuclide cineangiography during exercise. In this communication, we will illustrate the clinical uses of the technique with examples of data obtained from our patients with coronary artery disease.

METHODS

Cardiac scintigraphy is performed with subjects in the supine position at rest and during exercise as previously described (7). To perform this prodecure, human serum albumin labeled with 10 mCi of radioactive technetium (Tc-99m) is administered intravenously. After equilibration of the tracer in the blood pool, a conventional Anger camera (field of view = 25.4-cm diameter), equipped with a high-sensitivity parallel hole collimator, is oriented in the modified left anterior oblique position (1-3), to isolate the left ventricle in the field of view. Imaging is accomplished by the use of our previously described computed-based electrocardiographically-gated procedure (1-4) which has been modified to reduce data processing time and the interval required to achieve statistical reliability (5,6). The spatial resolution of this system is one centimeter as assessed by line spread function.

Data are collected and concurrently organized into a series of images (framing rate up to 100 frames/sec) residing in core and spanning the average cardiac cycle. While data are being acquired, these images can be displayed in rapid sequence, that is, in endless-loop flicker-free movie format. Thus, qualitative information regarding spatial and temporal variations of the cardiac chambers is immediately accessible. Visually interpretable information is produced within 30 seconds of the onset of data collection, and statistically reliable results within one to two minutes (5,6). Because of the rapidity of data collection, the procedure can be applied to studies performed during exercise, even in patients with coronary artery disease in whom exercise-induced ischemia and angina might preclude prolonged exercise and imaging (7,8) (Figs. 1 and 2).

EFFECT OF EXERCISE ON LEFT VENTRICULAR FUNCTION
CORONARY ARTERY DISEASE

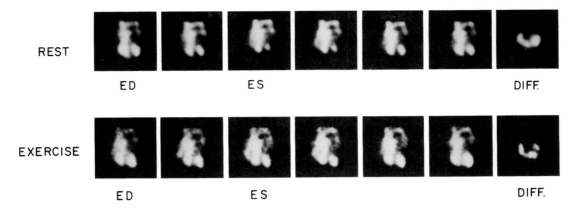

FIG. 1. Selected frames, in sequence, from a radionuclide cineangiogram taken in a patient with three-vessel coronary-artery disease at rest (upper) and during maximal exercise (lower). ED: end-diastolic frame; ES: end-systolic frame; DIFF: difference image (created by electronic subtraction of end-systolic images from end-diastolic image). (Reprinted, with permission, from Ref. 7.)

EFFECT OF EXERCISE ON LEFT VENTRICULAR FUNCTION
NORMAL

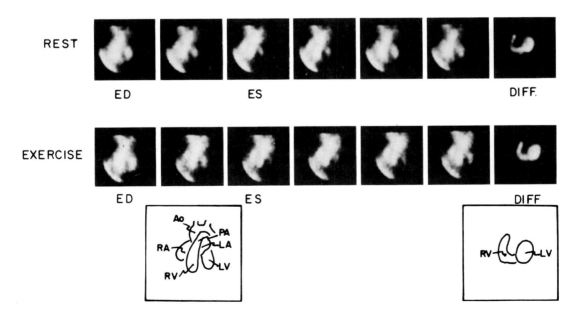

FIG. 2. Selected frames, in sequence, from a radionuclide cineangiogram taken in a normal subject at rest (upper) and during maximal exercise (lower). Ao: aorta; PA: pulmonary artery; RA: right atrium; RV: right ventricle; LA: left atrium; and LV: left ventricle. (Reprinted, with permission, from Ref. 7.)

While the cardiac images are being created, the computer simultaneously analyzes the acquired data to produce a time-activity curve with high (10-msec) temporal resolution (1-6) (Figure 3). Corrections for background activity are made as previously described (1-3). Since blood radioactivity is proportional to blood volume, after correction for background the time-activity curve in fact represents a measure of left ventricular volume versus time. Therefore, once the physician has identified the left ventricle ("region of interest") in the end-diastolic movie frame, quantitation of left ventricular volume change with time can be performed.

Unfortunately, although radioactive emissions are indeed proportional to volume, the proportionality constant is usually not known, and thus absolute volumes as yet cannot be determined. Two sets of factors determine the constant of proportionality between counts and volume: (a) factors associated with attenuation, detector efficiency and blood volume, and (b) factors associated with the amount and effective decay of the isotope. The former set of factors may be considered constant with time following a single injection of isotope. The latter set of factors are not constant with time, but over short intervals, their variation with time may be calculated. This calculation allows determination of relative, but not absolute, changes in end-diastolic volume or end-systolic volume as a function of time, and thus permits assessment of the effects of interventions (e.g., exercise) on these volumes.

The effective half-life of ^{99m}Tc-labelled albumin has been measured (15). Though the uncertainties in such measurements may be high, over short periods of time, large uncertainties in the effective half life cause only very small uncertainties in the change in volume. In our studies, imaging at rest and during exercise almost always is completed within 30 minutes in any one patient. Using a range of effective half lives of 3 to 5 hours (15) the half-life correction factor ranges from 0.89 to 0.93 (thus providing a 4% uncertainty) if rest and exercise are separated by 30 minutes. The correction factors, and inherent uncertainty, are smaller if, as is most common, the separation between studies is less than 30 minutes.

Statistically reliable information is obtained by summing the radioactivity in the ventricle during many beats. After each cardiac cycle the length of the RR interval is automatically examined to determine if it lies within a physician-selected temporal beat-length "window". Cycles falling outside this window are rejected to prevent distortion of the time-activity curve by premature beats. The movie can be similarly windowed. In a study of 39 patients, ejection fractions obtained by this method demonstrated excellent correlation with those obtained by contrast angiography with the patient at rest ($r = 0.92$, $p \leq .01$). Excellent interobserver agreement among three independent observers also was noted ($r = 0.95$, $p < .01$). In addition, ten studies performed at rest and during exercise were assessed twice by a single, blinded observer. Intervals between assessments of a single study ranged from 6 to 18 months. In no study was the second assessment more than five ejection fraction units (5%) different from the initial assessment, indicating excellent intraobserver reproducibility.

After the images and time-activity curves are obtained at rest, the subjects are asked to pedal a bicycle ergometer. A restraining harness is employed to prevent significant patient motion under the camera during exercise.

EFFECT OF EXERCISE ON
LEFT VENTRICULAR FUNCTION

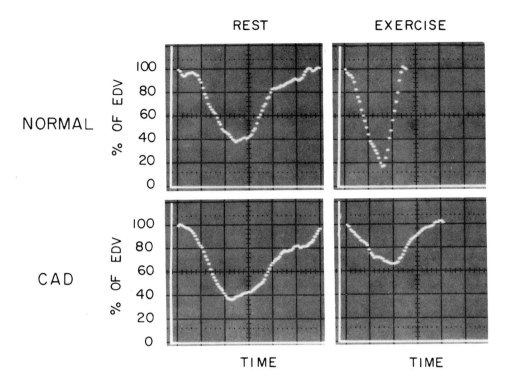

FIG. 3. Effect of exercise on left ventricular function—left ventricular time-activity curves from studies shown in Figs. 1 and 2. Note that ejection fraction (EDV-ESV/EDV) increases with exercise in the normal subject and decreases with exercise in the patient with coronary-artery disease (CAD). (Reprinted, with permission, from Ref. 7.)

Subjects exercise until limited by fatigue or by symptoms referable to their heart disease. Imaging can be undertaken throughout exercise with analysis performed only on the part of the record that is of clinical interest. However, in practice we usually begin imaging when the patient has reached ten beats per minute below the previously determined maximal heart rate. In the studies to be discussed, imaging continued for at least two minutes. In all studies, heart rate and blood pressure, obtained by arm cuff sphygmomanometry, are recorded.

When imaging is completed, left ventricular ejection fractions at rest and during exercise are determined automatically from the left ventricular time-activity curves (1-4). The computer-based movies are used in the qualitative visual assessment of regional left ventricular function at rest and during exercise. While it is possible to quantitate regional function with this technique by defining the region of interest as only part of the left ventricle, it is yet to be determined that such quantitation offers any clinically useful advantage over visual assessment in the detection of coronary artery disease.

In our studies movies usually are constructed from images obtained in the modified left anterior oblique (LAO) position. Therefore, function of the anteroseptal and anterolateral ventricular walls can be evaluated from the movie. Movie assessment of other surfaces of the heart can be achieved by imaging with the camera oriented in positions other than the LAO; however, in practice, we usually assess function of regions not at the border of the LAO silhouette by the use of count based "difference images", or "functional maps", created by subtracting the end-systolic image from the end-diastolic image, as previously described (2,3). In the resulting difference image (Figs. 1 and 2) the intensity (brightness) of each region of the image is proportional to the absolute change in radioactive emissions (volume) between diastole and systole in that region. Thus, in the LAO view a region of darkness located centrally in the difference image and surrounded by brighter regions (i.e., a non-edge-bordered defect) must represent either a posterobasal or an anterobasal region from which blood is not being ejected in as great a quantity as from surrounding regions. Abnormal regional function can be inferred with high specificity from this finding.

CLINICAL STUDIES

To evaluate the degree to which patient motion might alter the results of assessment of radionuclide images, nine studies were performed in normal volunteers with two cobalt line sources taped to their chests. Full width half maximum was determined at rest and during exercise (maximal load 200 watts, exceeding that achieved by any patient). Full-width half-maximum at rest (approximately 1 cm) was not significantly different from that noted during exercise, indicating that, while motion may occur during exercise, its magnitude does not exceed the spatial resolution of this system.

After this preliminary trial, we began our assessment of patients with heart disease. In our initial series, we studied 11 patients with arteriographically demonstrated coronary artery disease but with normal left ventricular regional and global function at rest as determined by contrast angiography. We found that during exercise each developed at least one region of left ventricular dysfunction, invariably in an area supplied by an artery with ≥ 50% stenosis (7). In addition, in these patients, global ejection fraction invariably fell during exercise as compared with rest.   In contrast, in 14 normal subjects, no regional dysfunction was present at rest or during exercise, and ejection fraction invariably rose with exercise.   The development of regional dysfunction during exercise is demonstrated in Figs. 1 and 2, which depict selected movie frames and difference images from studies in a normal subject and in a patient with three vessel coronary artery disease. The time-activity curves associated with these studies are depicted in Fig. 3.

In a more extensive series of 25 normal subjects and 47 consecutive patients with coronary artery disease (8) regional dysfunction invariably was noted during exercise, and ejection fraction fell from 48% at rest to 36% (p < .001) with exercise.   Though 30 patients had ejection fractions within the normal range (45% to 71%, average 57%) at rest, only one patient maintained an ejection fraction within the normal range during exercise.   All normal subjects increased ejection fraction during exercise (range = 55% to 93%, average 71%, p < .001 compared with normal subjects at rest and with patients with coronary artery disease during exercise).   Of note, no correlation was noted between patient age and ejection fraction at rest or exercise.   In addition, regional and global functional abnormalities were noted during exercise in all 14 of the 47 patients who did not develop angina during exercise (8). Three of these patients had no prior history suggestive of coronary artery disease.

These results indicate that radionuclide cineangiography during exercise is valuable in the diagnosis of coronary artery disease, even in the asymptomatic individual.   Moreover, these early results have been indistinguishable from the results of subsequent studies in more than 100 patients with coronary artery disease.

Although reduction in ejection fraction to subnormal levels during exercise is a non-specific concommitant of many forms of heart disease (9, 13, 14) regional dysfunction is seldom noted except in patients with coronary artery disease.   Therefore, we have used the presence of regional dysfunction as the criterion for the diagnosis of coronary artery disease.   Using this criterion, we have found that the radionuclide technique, which permits direct visualization of the heart, is significantly more sensitive in the detection of coronary artery disease than is the indirect exercise electrocardiographic procedure, and, in addition, is highly specific (10).

Because it permits assessment of the functional severity of coronary artery disease, radionuclide cineangiography is well suited to the evaluation of the efficacy of therapy in these patients.   To determine the value of the technique in the assessment of therapy, we studied 28 patients with coronary artery disease and 11 normal subjects before and after the administration of nitroglycerin (8).   While regional and global function during exercise in patients with coronary artery disease improved significantly after nitroglycerin (EF during exercise before nitroglycerin = 36%, after nitroglycerin = 48%, p < .001), the drug did not affect left ventricular function during exercise in normal subjects (8).   In a companion study, radionuclide cineangiography during exercise was able to demonstrate improvement in left ventricular function in a large group of patients with patent grafts following coronary artery bypass grafting (12).   Thus, the technique has proven useful in the evaluation of therapy.

Radionuclide cineangiography has been applied to the evaluation of over 400 patients with cardiac abnormalities other than coronary artery disease. The value of such studies is exemplified by our findings in patients with aortic regurgitation (9,11). In this group, abnormal left ventricular function during exercise has been demonstrated in asymptomatic patients with normal function at rest. Such findings are expected to be of great clinical value in the determination of the appropriate timing of operation, and a prospective study now is underway to evaluate the prognostic significance of the radionuclide findings. The technique also has been found efficacious in the assessment of the results of aortic valve replacement in patients with aortic regurgitation (11).

DISCUSSION

Our data indicate that radionuclide cineangiography during exercise has important clinical value. However, when the technique first was introduced (7), concern was expressed regarding the validity of data obtained during exercise, since exercise can cause patient movement beneath the Anger camera. Therefore, it might be anticipated that studies during exercise could result in distorted images which might obscure wall motion and cause difficulty in interpretation. Fortunately, as discussed elsewhere (8), this is not a practical problem when the technique is used qualitatively to estimate contractile function of large regions of the left ventricle. That this is true is indicated by 1) the accuracy of regional function alalysis with this technique in indicating the presence or absence of coronary artery disease in a given patient (that is, in separating normal from abnormal (7,8)), and 2) the very good correlation between the presence of a regional abnormality during exercise and the presence of a ≥ 50% stenosis of the coronary artery supplying this region, with no false positives having been noted (7).

There are several explanations for the utility of the technique in providing interpretable information during exercise. However, even when performed at rest, radionuclide angiographic procedures inherently have relatively poor spatial resolution (generally approximately 1 cm full width half maximum). Despite this limitation, regional function abnormalities present at rest during radionuclide angiography have been demonstrated by several authors (16,17) to correlate well with wall motion abnormalities observed during contrast angiography. Radionuclide techniques permit assessment of regional function despite such relatively limited spatial resolution because, while their display format appears to be two-dimensional, in fact count-based radionuclide imaging permits visual perception of changes in three-dimensional volume, with volume being proportional to the brightness of the image in any region. Therefore, perception of changes in the motion of the edge of the cardiac silhouette is markedly enhanced by perception of changes in volume (brightness) of the region adjacent to the edge. Moreover, small changes in wall motion cause relatively larger changes in regional volume.

Thus, some motion (up to 1 cm) may be tolerated without perceptible reduction in the change in relative intensity of radioactive emissions in a given region during the cardiac cycle. Even greater motion may not preclude visual perception of abnormalities in the combination of edge motion plus regional volume change during the cardiac cycle. Nonetheless, to limit such motion we use a restrictive harness system to mimimize patient movement both in the cephalad-caudad direction and in the lateral direction. Such maneuvers are successful in limiting motion as demonstrated by our assessment of line spread function in normal volunteers. Moreover, we do not attempt to resolve the location of abnormalities with any great precision. For example, in the LAO view, the anteroseptal region includes that portion of the left ventricular silhouette to the left of the midline and the anterolateral region includes that portion of the left ventricular silhouette to the right of the midline.

In addition, the ability to perceive abnormal motion is enhanced by the use of the movie display format. Since fixed background structures (liver, spleen, great vessels) are available as reference points, the motion of the heart relative to these structures can be assessed visually even if the entire body moves slightly. Such assessment would be difficult or impossible with still frame display.

Finally, determination of a count-based ejection fraction does not depend upon precise definition of left ventricular boundaries. As long as the left ventricle is separated from other cardiac structures, as it is in the modified left anterior oblique view (30 to 40 degrees left anterior oblique position, 15 degrees caudad modification), it is possible to define a "region of interest" containing the entire left ventricle throughout the cardiac cycle, but which contains no other cardiac chamber.

During the cardiac cycle, the change in radioactive emissions within this region must be due only to movement of blood into and out of the left ventricle. Ventricular geometry, or movement of the ventricle within the region of interest, does not affect the change in radioactive emissions and therefore does not affect the ejection fraction determined by this technique. Moreover, in practice, once again, the changes in ejection fraction from rest to exercise in normal subjects were significantly different from the changes in patients with heart disease. Of note, there is corroborative evidence regarding the development of wall motion abnormalities and of ejection fraction abnormalities during exercise from the work of Sharma, who found results similar to ours when he used contrast ventriculography to assess patients with coronary artery disease (18).

CONCLUSION

Our data indicate that non-invasive radionuclide cineangiography is a simple and apparently sensitive technique permitting determination of regional and global left ventricular function both at rest and during exercise. It is useful in the diagnosis of coronary artery disease, in assessment of the functional severity of disease and of the efficacy of therapy in patients with various cardiac abnormalities, and it may provide information of prognostic importance to aid in the optimal timing of therapy. We believe, therefore, that this computer-based technique, the result of several years of preclinical research by a team of radiation physicists, computer scientists and clinicians, is now a valuable clinical tool in the evaluation of patients with heart disease.

ACKNOWLEDGEMENTS

We gratefully acknowledge the invaluable technical assistance of Bonnie Mack, B.S., and Susan Farkas, B.A., in the performance of these studies.

REFERENCES

1.   Green MV, Ostrow HG, Douglas MA, et al: High temporal resolution EGC-gated scintigraphic angiocardiography. J Nuc Med 16: 95-98, 1975.

2.   Green MV, Bacharach SL, Douglas MA, et al: The measurement of left ventricular function and the detection of wall motion abnormalities with high temporal resolution ECG-gated scintigraphic angiocardiography. IEEE Transac Nuclear Sci NS23: 1257-1263, 1976.

3.   Green MV, Bailey JJ, Ostrow HG, et al: Computerized ECG-gated radionuclide angiocardiography. A non-invasive method for determining left ventricular volumes and focal myocardial dyskinesia. Computers in Cardiology, Rotterdam, The Netherlands. Proceedings of the IEEE Computer Society, 1975, pp 137-141.

4.   Douglas MA, Ostrow HG, Green MV, et al: A computer processing system for ECG-gated radioisotope angiography of the human heart. Computers Biomed Res 9: 133-142, 1976.

5.   Bacharach SL, Green MV, Borer JS, et al: A real-time system for multi-image gated cardiac studies. J Nuc Med 18: 79-84, 1977.

6.   Bacharach SL, Green MV, Borer JS, et al: Real-time scintigraphic cineangiography. Computers in Cardiology, Proceedings of the IEEE Computer Society, St. Louis, Missouri, 1976, pp 45-48.

7.   Borer JS, Bacharach SL, Green MV, et al: Application of real-time radionuclide cineangiography in the non-invasive evaluation of global and regional left ventricular function at rest and during exercise in patients with coronary artery disease. New Engl J Med 296: 839-844, 1977.

8.   Borer JS, Bacharach SL, Green MV, et al: Effect of nitroglycerin on exercise-induced abnormalities of left ventricular regional function and ejection fraction in coronary artery disease: Assessment by radionuclide cineangiography in symptomatic and asymptomatic patients. Circulation, in press (February, 1978).

9.   Borer JS, Bacharach SL, Green MV, et al: Exercise-induced left ventricular dysfunction in symptomatic and asymptomatic patients with severe aortic regurgitation assessed by radionuclide cineangiography. Am J Cardiol 39: 284, 1977 (Abs).

10.   Borer JS, Kent KM, Bacharach SL, et al: Accuracy of radionuclide cineangiography in detecting coronary artery disease: Comparison with exercise electrocardiography. Circulation 56: Suppl III: III-33, 1977 (Abs).

11.   Borer JS, Bacharach SL, Green MV, et al: Left ventricular function during exercise before and after aortic valve replacement. Circulation 56: Suppl III: III-28, 1977 (Abs).

12.   Kent KM, Borer JS, Green MV, et al: Effects of coronary artery bypass operation on global and regional left ventricular function during exercise. Clinical Research 25: 230A, 1977 (Abs).

13. Borer JS, Bacharach SL, Green MV, et al: Left ventricular function in aortic stenosis: Response to exercise and effects of operation. Am J Cardiol, in press (Abs).

14. Borer JS, Bacharach SL, Green MV, et al: Obstructive vs nonobstructive asymmetric septal hypertrophy: Differences in left ventricular function with exercise. Am J Cardiol, in press (Abs).

15. Herbert RJT, Hibbard BM, Sheppard MA: Metabolic behavior and radiation dosimetry of ^{99m}Tc-albumin in pregnancy. J Nuc Med 10: 224-232, 1969.

16. Zaret BL, Strauss HW, Hurley PJ, et al: A scintiphotographic method for detecting regional ventricular dysfunction in man. N Engl J Med 284: 1165-1170, 1971.

17. Salel AF, Berman DS, DeNardo GL, et al: Radionuclide assessment of nitroglycerin influence on abnormal left ventricular segmental contraction in patients with coronary heart disease. Circulation 53: 975-982, 1976.

18. Sharma B, Goodwin JF, Raphael MJ, et al: Left ventricular angiography on exercise: A new method of assessing left ventricular function in ischaemic heart disease. Br Heart J 38: 59-70, 1976.

EXERCISE STRESS FIRST-PASS RADIONUCLIDE LEFT VENTRICULAR FUNCTION (EJECTION FRACTION AND SEGMENTAL WALL MOTION)

James A. Jengo, J. Michael Uszler, Richard Conant,
Marianne Brizendine and Ismael Mena

Harbor General Hospital
Divisions of Cardiology and Nuclear Medicine
Torrance, Ca. 90509

ABSTRACT

The significance of coronary arterial obstruction is dependent upon its effect on left ventricular function. Exercise induced stress is a commonly accepted method for provoking myocardial ischemia in asymptomatic patients with coronary artery disease. The purpose of this study was to develop a noninvasive, rapid technique for determining left ventricular function both at rest and during maximal upright exercise stress. In the normal group the ejection fraction significantly increased from rest to exercise: $0.65 \pm .03$ to $0.81 \pm .03$ (m ± SEM) $p < .005$, as did segmental wall motion. In the coronary artery disease group the ejection fraction either did not change or decreased during exercise: $0.59 \pm .07$ to $0.42 \pm .06$ ($p < .005$). Segmental wall motion significantly decreased in the area(s) supplied by the stenosed arteries. Therefore, this technique provides the rapid noninvasive evaluation of left ventricular function during maximal upright exercise; the functional separation of normal subjects from those with significant coronary artery disease; and localization of the area of ischemic dysfunction.

INTRODUCTION

The true significance of coronary arterial narrowing is dependent upon its effect on left ventricular function. Currently available non-invasive techniques for evaluation of left ventricular function are used only during the resting state. Since angiographically demonstrable severe coronary artery disease does not necessarily result in myocardial ischemia and its consequent left ventricular dysfunction at rest (1, 2, 3), exercise induced stress is a commonly used and accepted method for provoking myocardial ischemia in patients with coronary artery disease. Currently available radionuclide techniques permit the evaluation of left ventricular function at rest or with moderate supine exercise, but do not achieve the functional ideal of maximal upright exercise stress (4).

At present contrast angiography is the "gold standard" in the evaluation of left ventricular function. However exercise stress induced changes in left ventricular function are not commonly evaluated because of the difficulty of exercising the supine patient and the myocardial depressent effects of repeated injections of contrast material.

The purpose of this study was to develop a noninvasive, rapid technique for the determination of left ventricular ejection fraction and segmental wall motion both at rest and during maximal upright exercise stress. The technique of first-pass radionuclide angiography was applied before and during maximal upright bicycle stress in subjects with normal or angiographically proven nonsignificantly stenosed coronary arteries, and in those with angiographically proven significant coronary artery disease.

EXERCISE PROTOCOL

To perform studies at the time of exercising the subject requires overcoming the problem of patient motion. To accomplish this the exercise is performed with the subject facing the gamma scintillation camera detector (mobile Ohio-Nuclear Sigma 410, with high-sensitivity collimator) in the 30 degree RAO projection while seated on a bicycle ergometer. Prior to the start of the exercise an intravenous line and pertinent cardiac monitoring equipment are attached to the subject as for a routine exercise electrocardiographic stress test. A foam rubber wedge is placed at the precordial area to keep the subject in the RAO projection. The subject is then held to the detector and the wedge by a strap around his back and connected at each of its ends to the camera detector. In addition the subject grasps with his two arms the arms of the detector gantry. The mobile camera detector gantry has a small amount of free movement such that it moves with the patient while he pedals the bicycle. In this way the patient is motionless relative to the detector because the patient motion is transferred to the camera gantry itself. At the time of the subject's maximal stress a 30-second gamma camera acquisition is obtained after a bolus of radionuclide (15 millicuries of 99mTc pertechnetate) is flushed into an antecubital vein. Each subject was previously studied at rest with similar injection technique.

DATA ACQUISITION AND HANDLING

The list mode data was simultaneously recorded on the camera's high speed (75 ips) magnetic tape drive and also simultaneously acquired on the disc of a mini-computer system (Informatek Simis-3) for calculation of ejection fraction and determination of segmental wall motion.

The study is first reviewed for motion artifact using the persistence mode on the mini-computer display. Ejection fraction was calculated from a background-corrected left ventricular time/activity curve framed with a dt of 40 milliseconds. Segmental wall motion was subsequently determined from end-diastolic and end-systolic frames (selected from the left ventricular volume curve) using a modified second derivative approach (5).

RESULTS

In the control group of patients (4 normals and 4 patients with less than 50% coronary artery occlusion) the ejection fraction significantly increased from rest to exercise: $0.65 \pm .03$ to $0.81 \pm .03$ (m ± SEM), $p < .005$. Segmental wall motion measured over the 2 anterior and 2 inferoposterior segments was also uniformly increased during exercise.

In the group of 11subjects with a history of angina and angiographically proven significant coronary artery disease (>75% occlusion) the ejection fraction did not change in 3 patients, and significantly decreased in the remaining : 0.59 ± 0.07 to 0.42 ± 0.06, $p < .005$. In all subjects segmental wall motion significantly decreased in the area(s) supplied by the stenosed coronary arteries (Table 1, Figs. 1 and 2).

DISCUSSION

Ejection fraction is a sensitive indicator of global left ventricular function, but may not reveal changes in regional contractility. Changes in segmental wall motion have been shown to be very sensitive indicators of regional left ventricular function (6). Of note, in this study it was seen that the ejection fraction at rest was not significantly different in the subjects with normal or significantly stenosed coronary arteries.

In those patients with angiographically significant coronary artery disease, both regional and global decreases in left ventricular function became apparent during exercise stress. Therefore in a significant proportion of patients with severe coronary artery disease, left ventricular functional impairment could only be demonstrated during exercise stress.

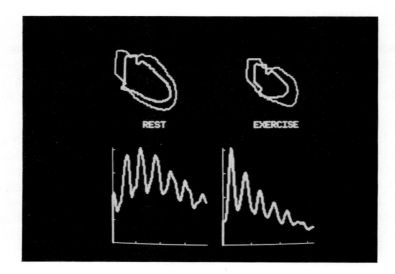

FIG. 1. Examples of a normal resting and exercise angiocardiogram. The left panels represent segmental wall motion in RAO projection. Uniform wall motion can be seen throughout the entire ventricle. The ejection fraction in this patient was normal. In the right panel the response to this patient's exercise is seen. It can be seen that end-diastolic volume is decreased and wall motion improved uniformly throughout the ventricle. Ejection fraction increased.

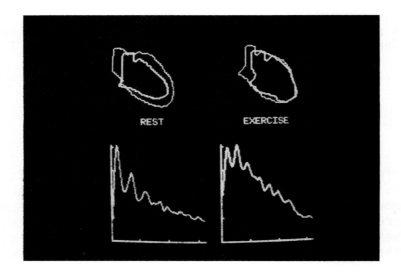

FIG. 2. Resting and exercise angiocardiograms in a patient with significant coronary artery disease. The left panel demonstrates the resting radionuclide angiocardiogram and shows normal uniform wall motion at rest with normal ejection fraction. However, the right panel demonstrates this patient's response to exercise. It can be seen that the ejection fraction falls markedly and anteroapical akinesis becomes manifest.

TABLE 1. CORONARY ARTERY DISEASE

Patient	Heart Rate	EXERCISE STRESS Chest Pain	EXERCISE STRESS ST Depression	EJECTION FRACTION Rest	EJECTION FRACTION Exercise	SEGMENTAL WALL MOTION REST AB	REST AA	REST IA	REST IB	EXERCISE AB	EXERCISE AA	EXERCISE IA	EXERCISE IB
1	125	-	+	60	53	2+	2+	1+	2+	3+	3+	3+	3+
2	145	+	-	80	58	3+	3+	3+	3+	1+	1+	1+	1+
3	120	+	-	73	54	3+	3+	3+	3+	1+	0	1+	2+
4	148	+	-	29	29	1+	1+	0	1+	1+	0	0	2+
5	130	-	-	47	39	2+	2+	1+	2+	2+	2+	0	1+
6	105	+	+	53	53	2+	1+	2+	2+	1+	1+	2+	2+
7	140	-	-	58	44	2+	2+	2+	2+	2+	2+	2+	1+
8	103	+	+	71	36	2+	2+	1+	1+	2+	2+	0	0
9	159	-	-	44	32	1+	0	0	2+	0	1-	0	1+
10	147	-	-	50	50	3+	2+	2+	2+	3+	2+	2+	2+
11	152	+	+	68	44	2+	0	3+	3+	3+	1-	2+	3+

+: present; -: absent; AB: anterobasal; AA: anteroapical; IA: inferoapical; IB: inferobasal; 1-: dyskinetic; 0: akinetic; 1+: hypokinetic; 2+: normal; 3+: hyperkinetic

Therefore the technique of first pass radionuclide stress angiography provides: 1) a rapid noninvasive means of evaluating left ventricular function during maximal upright exercise stress; 2) the functional separation of subjects with significant obstructive coronary artery disease; 3) localization of the area of ischemic dysfunction.

ACKNOWLEDGEMENTS

The authors would like to thank Dr. Thomas Nelson and Mr. Sheldon Chelsy for their technical expertise and Ms. Ann Lubahn for the typing of this manuscript.

REFERENCES

1.   Selzer A.,Cohn K: Asymptomatic coronary artery disease and coronary bypass surgery. Am.J. Cardiol. 39:614, 1977.

2.   Tennant R, Wiggers CJ: The effect of coronary occlusion on myocardial contractions. Am. J. Physiol. 112:351, 1935.

3.   Sharma B, Goodwin JF, Raphael MJ, Steiner RE, Rainbow RG, Taylor SH: Left ventricular angiography on exercise: A new method of assessing left ventricular function in ischemic heart disease. British Heart Journal 38:59, 1976.

4.   Borer JS, Bacharach SL, Green MY, et al: Real-time radionuclide cineangiography in the non-invasive evaluation of global and regional left ventricular function at rest and during exercise in patients with coronary-artery disease. N. Engl. J. Med. 296: 839, 1977.

5.   Jengo JA, Mena I, Blaufuss A, Criley JM: Evaluation of left ventricular function (Ejection fraction and segmental wall motion) by single pass radioisotope angiography. Circulation (in press) February 1978.

6.   Herman MD, Heinle RA, Klein MD, Gorlin R: Localized disorders in myocardial contraction: Asynergy and its role in congestive heart failure. N. Engl. J. Med. 277:222, 1967.

INITIAL EXPERIENCE WITH SIMULTANEOUS DUAL PROJECTION RADIONUCLIDE VENTRICULOGRAPHY

Stewart M. Spies, Jose M. Cuevas and Thomas W. Ryerson

Northwestern University Medical School
Department of Radiology
Chicago, Illinois 60611

The growing importance of radioisotopes in evaluation of cardiovascular disease has resulted in a variety of recent innovations and refinements which have improved the accuracy of these techniques. The initial experience with a new collimator system which enables simultaneous acquisition of images of the cardiac blood pool in two projections is described. Measurements of sensitivity and spatial resolution confirm the "general purpose" (medium sensitivity - medium resolution) nature of the device. Clinical evaluation comparing results with the dual collimator and a high resolution parallel hole collimator indicated close agreement with regard to ejection fraction determination and reasonably close agreement with regard to segmental wall motion. The advantages and disadvantages of dual projection collimation are discussed.

INTRODUCTION

Recent advances in radiopharmaceuticals and instrumentation, along with improved implementation of data processing techniques, have resulted in a revolution in nuclear cardiology: of particular importance is the use of radioisotopic procedures to evaluate global and regional left ventricular function. Such techniques offer the clinician a noninvasive approach to evaluation of cardiac dynamics in patients with a wide spectrum of clinical disorders including valvular heart disease, coronary artery disease, cardiomyopathy and congenital heart disease. Three fundamental approaches have been used to obtain this functional information. The first approach is the so-called "first pass" method which relies on analysis of images obtained during the first transit through the heart of a bolus of activity injected into the venous system, usually through an arm vein ([1]). The second method, equilibrium gated analysis, employs an intravascular tracer imaged at equilibrium with creation of an average cardiac cycle image through synchronization of image collection with the patient's electrocardiogram ([2]). The third method, not currently in wide use, employs probe data without imaging to yield quantitative information about global left ventricular function ([3]).

Presently the first two techniques, which rely on data obtained from gamma camera images, are most often employed. Because of the importance of assessing regional wall motion, in addition to total left ventricular ejection fraction, the use of more than one projection offers an advantage over single projection studies since more than one view is required to adequately evaluate all segments of the left ventricular myocardium. Using conventional imaging equipment, multiple projections would require multiple injections with the first transit method, or repositioning and additional data acquisition with the equilibrium gated techniques.

We will report our initial experience with a new collimator developed for use with conventional gamma camera systems, which simultaneously provides two projections of the cardiac blood pool activity.

DESCRIPTION OF COLLIMATOR

The dual projection collimator is a lead collimator consisting of 6100 parallel rectangular channels divided into two groups. In the Y direction, the holes of each group are parallel, but in the X direction the holes of one group start toward the holes of the opposite group, resulting in a 60-degree angle between projections of the two sections of the collimator. This in effect results in two separate collimation systems which, when placed flat against a patient's chest, will simultaneously provide a 30-degree right anterior oblique and a 30-degree left anterior oblique projection. The collimator is designed for photon energies up to 200 kev, and was equipped with a mounting ring which permitted it to be attached to the detector of a Picker 4/15 large field of view camera. Some collimator performance characteristics are summarized in Tables 1 and 2.

TABLE 1.   SENSITIVITY COMPARISON (^{99m}Tc)

Dual Collimator

Right Side	430 cpm/ μCi
Left Side	430 cpm/ μCi
Both Sides	870 cpm/ μCi

Conventional Collimators

Ultrafine (HR)	258 cpm/ μCi
Tc Dynamic (HS)	1166 cpm/ μCi
Tc LEAP	474 cpm/ μCi

TABLE 2.   SPATIAL RESOLUTION, DUAL PROJECTION COLLIMATOR (^{99m}Tc)

Source-to-Collimator Distance (cm)	FWHM (A)[*] (cm)	FWHM (B)[*]
0.0	0.31	
2.5	0.91	
5.0	1.17	
7.5	1.42	1.42
10.0	1.62	1.69
12.5	1.99	1.79
15.0	2.25	2.32

[*] A and B are the two projections seen by the dual projection collimator. Projection B is not seen until source-to-collimator distance is 7.5 cm.

CLINICAL STUDIES

Clinical studies consisted of comparison of data obtained while using the dual projection collimator with data obtained using a conventional collimator. All patients were studied with the following protocol:

1. An intravascular radiopharmaceutical was obtained by the method of in vivo erythrocyte labeling (4).

2. Equilibrium gated images were obtained employing the dual projection collimator and Picker 4/15 camera. The camera was interfaced to a PDP 11/34 minicomputer with 32K words of MOS memory and 4.8 megabytes of cartridge disc storage. The patient's electrocardiogram was processed by a peak detect circuit and and R wave coincidence pulses were supplied to the computer through a separate I/O port. Data were collected in frame mode as 12 core-resident images, each 64x64x8 bits, and each representing 1/12 of an average cardiac cycle. When an overflow occurred in any byte-mode image, the images were recorded on a disc in word mode, and a new set of core-resident images begun. Data collection was terminated when a predetermined number of total study counts was achieved, generally 16 million events. Arrhythmia detection software rejected cycles outside user defined limits. By positioning the collimator flat against the supine patient, 30-degree LAO and 30-degree RAO projections, each containing approximately 8 million events, were obtained.

3. Immediately following the simultaneous images described above, the patient was placed beneath a mobile scintillation camera (Searle LEM or Picker Dynamo) equipped with a high resolution collimator, and images were obtained in the 30-degree RAO, 30-degree LAO and 60-degree LAO projections (the standard protocol for this laboratory). The data acquisition was performed on the same system in an identical fashion to that described for the dual projection collimator.

DATA ANALYSIS

The data obtained using the dual projection collimator and the data obtained from the corresponding separate images (30^0 LAO and 30^{0}RAO) obtained using the conventional high resolution collimator in each patient were analyzed and compared as follows.

A qualitative evaluation of segmental wall motion was performed by creating a loop of images, each representing approximately 10% of an average cardiac cycle, and displaying them in a "cine" mode. For the purpose of this dynamic display the images were interpolated to 128x128 matrices, and a play back rate of approximately 10 frames/second was employed. The regions of the intraventricular septum, inferior wall apex, anterior wall, anterolateral wall, and posterolateral wall were examined for each image from each collimator. The results of this analysis are summarized in Figure 1.

Quantitative analysis of global left ventricular function was performed for each patient using the 30-degree LAO projection from the dual projection collimator and the 30-degree LAO projection data from the conventional collimator. The data analysis protocol consisted of assigning a region of interest manually to enclose the left ventricle, and assigning a background region lateral to the left ventricle. These regions were then used to generate a background-subtracted left ventricular volume curve for each collimator. From the curve the left ventricular ejection fraction and left ventricular ejection velocity were computed, the latter being obtained by a least squares fit of the downslope of the volume curve. Figures 2 and 3 show representative region assignments in one patient and Figures 4 and 5 show the corresponding volume curves and least squares fit used in obtaining the left ventricular functional parameters.

The results of quantitative analysis of ventricular function in six patients, using both the dual projection and conventional collimators, are summarized in Table 3.   The correlation coefficient of 0.94 indicates close agreement between the two methods, although linear regression analysis confirms that the ejection fraction obtained using the dual projection collimator was consistently lower than that obtained by conventional collimation.

Because the data collection matrix was the same for both collimators (64x64), the calibrated pixel size was necessarily larger for the dual collimator. The region of interest assignment was somewhat less accurate, as can be seen from examining the number of pixels comprising the left ventricular region in each patient, summarized in Table 4.

DISCUSSION AND SUMMARY

As with all collimation systems in nuclear medicine, the choice between dual projection collimation and conventional high-resolution collimation for isotope ventriculography is a matter of compromises. The spatial resolution and sensitivity of the dual projection collimator are roughly similar to those of a general purpose collimator. The improved spatial resolution did allow for somewhat better depiction of segmental wall motion using a conventional high-resolution collimator, although in only one of six patients was a wall motion abnormality missed by the dual collimator. It must be pointed out that since the conventional collimators employed were used on high-resolution cameras with 25 cm crystals and the dual collimator used on a 40 cm crystal, rigid quantitative comparison of these results is not valid. The close agreement in ejection fraction determinations suggest that either collimator is satisfactory for quantitating left ventricular function.

Segmental Wall Motion   (N = 6)

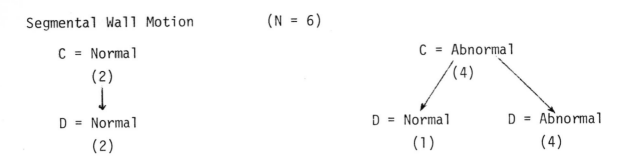

C = Normal   C = Abnormal
    (2)   (4)

D = Normal   D = Normal   D = Abnormal
    (2)   (1)   (4)

FIG. 1. Results of segmental wall motion analysis. (C = conventional collimator; D = dual projection collimator.)

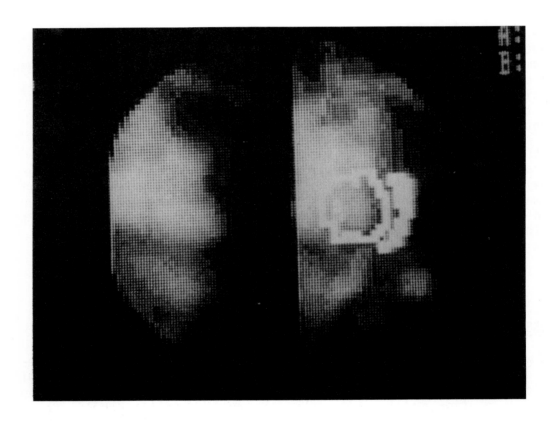

FIG. 2. Region of interest assignment for dual collimator.

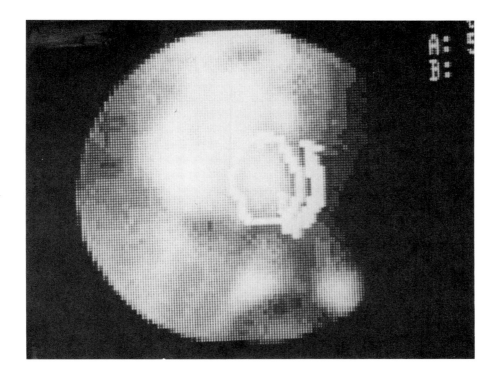

FIG. 3. Region of interest assignment for conventional collimator.

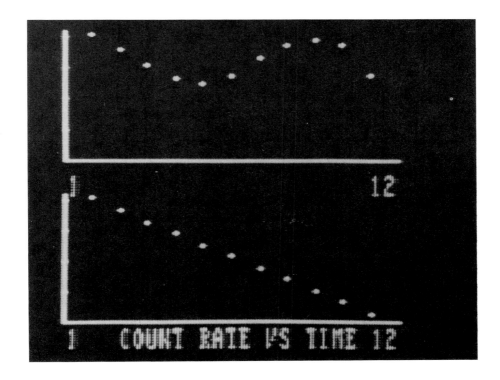

FIG. 4. Left ventricular volume curve and ejection velocity least squares fit for dual collimator.

TABLE 3.   LV EJECTION FRACTION

Dual Projection	Conventional
18	23
40	54
50	64
54	60
22	28
37	42

R = 0.94

Slope = 1.14

Intercept = 3.1

TABLE 4.   NUMBER OF MATRIX ELEMENTS COMPRISING LV REGION

Dual Projection (D)	Conventional (C)	D/C
323	594	.54
113	229	.49
104	193	.54
101	198	.52
186	397	.47
132	280	.47

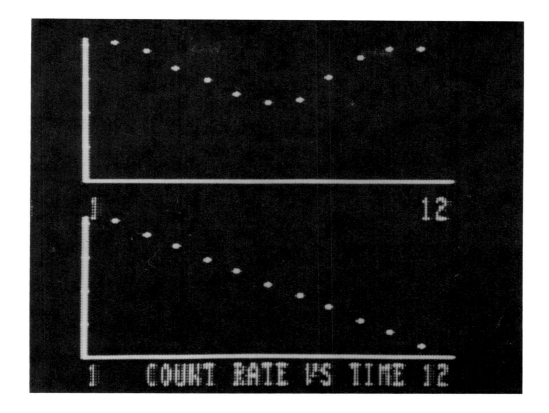

FIG. 5. Left ventricular volume curve and ejection velocity least squares fit for conventional collimator.

Certain observations can be made on the basis of this preliminary evaluation. There are several disadvantages to the use of the dual projection collimator for cardiac studies. The collimator tends to make inefficient use of the acquisition matrix when using a large field of view camera. Hardware zooming by increasing ADC gains may not be practical unless performed only along one axis. The spatial resolution of the system evaluated may not be sufficient to identify subtle wall motion abnormalities within the detection range of conventional high resolution collimators. Finally, accurate region of interest assignment is somewhat more difficult due to the relative increase in calibrated pixel size.

On the other hand, there are several advantages favoring the use of dual projection collimation. The collimator allows one to acquire two projections during a first transit study using a single injection. The design allows the collimator to rest flat against the patient's chest, after the fashion of other "slant hole" collimators. The increased sensitivity allows some reduction in data acquisition time. Of special interest is the application of the dual projection system to exercise gated studies, where patient cooperation and endurance may not allow for two projections using conventional means. Also of importance is that no changes need be made in current data analysis software both in exhibiting cine displays and in quantitating ventricular parameters. Finally, the dual projection collimator may be applied to a variety of other cardiac and non-cardiac imaging procedures.

REFERENCES

1. Marshall RL, Freedman AS, Berger HJ et al: Left ventricular contrac-
    tility as assessed by normalized ejection velocity utilizing quanti-
    tative radionuclide angiocardiography and a computerized multi-crystal
    scintillation camera. J Nucl Med 17:566, 1976.

2. Borer JS, Bacharach SL, Green MV et al: Rest-time radionuclide cine-
    angiography. The noninvasive evaluation of global and regional left
    ventricular function at rest and during exercise in patients with
    coronary artery disease. N Eng J Med 296:839-844, 1977.

3. Bacharach SL, Green MV, Borer JS et al: ECG-gated scintillation
    probe measurement of left ventricular function. J Nucl Med 18:
    1176-1183, 1977.

4. Pavel DG, Zimmar AM and Patterson VN: In vivo labeling of red blood
    cells with ^{99m}Tc: A new approach to blood pool visualization.
    J Nucl Med 18:305-308, 1977.

FIRST-PASS RADIONUCLIDE ANGIOCARDIOGRAPHY FOR EVALUATION OF RIGHT AND LEFT VENTRICULAR PERFORMANCE: COMPUTER APPLICATIONS AND TECHNICAL CONSIDERATIONS

Harvey J. Berger, M. D.
Alexander Gottschalk, M. D.
Barry L. Zaret, M. D.*

Cardiology Section, Department of Internal Medicine
Nuclear Medicine Section, Department of Diagnostic Radiology
Yale University School of Medicine, New Haven, Connecticut 06510

ABSTRACT

First-pass radionuclide angiocardiography permits rapid noninvasive assessment of left and right ventricular performance. Left ventricular ejection fraction, mean normalized ejection rate, and regional wall motion, as well as right ventricular ejection fraction are obtained from analysis of regional time-activity curves. These techniques are free of the geometric assumptions inherent in conventional volume analysis. The anatomic and temporal separation of radioactivity within the ventricles during the first transit of the bolus through the central circulation allows combined evaluation of right and left ventricular function from a single study. Because data accumulation requires less than 20 seconds, this approach is ideally suited for assessment of rapidly changing physiologic states such as exercise.

Supported in part by NHLBI Contract N01HV52977 and NHLBI Grant R01HL21690-01

*Established Investigator of the American Heart Association

BACKGROUND

Quantitative first-pass radionuclide angiocardiography allows rapid non-invasive evaluation of global and regional ventricular performance. Indices of right and left ventricular function are derived directly from the high frequency components of regional time-activity curves obtained during the first transit of the radiotracer through the central circulation. Complete mixing of the bolus with blood is assumed to have occurred by the time the radionuclide has entered the right ventricle, such that changes in radioactivity reflect proportional changes in chamber volume. These methods are free of the geometric assumptions inherent in conventional volume analysis based upon intracavitary dimensions and planimetered areas used in contrast angiography and M-mode echocardiography. Because of the anatomic and temporal separation of the radionuclide bolus within each of the ventricles, first-pass radionuclide angiocardiography is ideal for evaluation of both right and left ventricular function from a single study.

The original quantitative studies of ventricular performance were reported in 1972 by Van Dyke et al (1) and Weber et al (2). They applied simple computer processing techniques to analysis of the first-pass angiocardiogram obtained with a conventional single crystal camera and found that the high frequency components of the left ventricular time-activity curve could be evaluated on a beat-to-beat basis, providing data on ejection fraction, an established parameter of left ventricular performance. Van Dyke et al (1) also noted that ejection fraction calculated directly from the uncorrected time-activity curve was consistently lower than that obtained with contrast angiography, even in normal subjects without regional abnormalities. Their studies pointed out the necessity of accounting for the contribution of radioactivity originating from background regions surrounding and underlying the left ventricular region of interest. In their studies, two regions of interest were identified, the end-diastolic left ventricular image and a ring around the entire left ventricle representing background. Time-activity curves were generated from each region, and after subtracting the background curve from the left ventricular time-activity curve, ejection fraction was calculated directly from the fractional fall in counts from end-diastole to end-systole over several beats. Since these original studies, several investigators have proposed modifications of this conceptual approach. All reported studies have demonstrated that this technique provides accurate data concerning left ventricular performance (3-6).

INSTRUMENTATION

The validity of the first-pass technique is dependent upon attaining sufficiently high count rates to minimize statistical uncertainty of radionuclide data. The deadtime or time required to process electronic events limits the maximal number of counts that a camera or computer system can accumulate. Assuming that spatial resolution does not deteriorate at higher count rates, a short deadtime is highly desirable. A long deadtime may cause dynamic flow data to become distorted. Most single crystal gamma cameras function with a deadtime of about five to twelve μsec and thus are limited in the maximal number of counts that can be recorded without distortion or loss of data (7). This is of particular importance in evaluating first transit studies of cardiac performance. In studies obtained with most single crystal scintillation cameras, the maximal end-diastolic count rate in the left ventricular region of interest is limited and often makes analysis of the data difficult. This problem prompted Schelbert et al (3) to use a root mean square transformation of the original time-activity curve in order to increase the statistical reliability of their data.

An alternative approach, which has been used in our laboratory (6,8) is the development of techniques applicable to the computerized multicrystal scintillation camera, a system with an extremely short deadtime. The detector of this instrument consists of a mosaic of 294 individual crystals arranged in a rectangular array of 14 columns and 21 rows. The crystals are coupled optically to 35 photomultiplier tubes by a complex light piping assembly. An individual scintillation occurring in a crystal generates a pulse in two tubes, defining the exact spatial location of the event. The output of the phototubes is amplified and subjected to pulse height analysis. Anti-coincidence circuits eliminate pulses arising simultaneously in more than one crystal. Pulses are stored as digital data in a solid-state buffer memory, allowing high speed storage of data during accumulation. Simultaneously, data are transfered from the memory to the disc by the computer system. The field of view of each crystal is limited by a single tapered hole provided by a lead collimator with 294 individual aligned holes. This allows the system to acquire data at rates up to approximately 250,000 counts/second without saturating the detector or introducing errors in the position pulses. Thus, the multicrystal camera has an effective deadtime of approximately two μsec. This provides high temporal resolution and is ideally suited for high count rate, first-pass cardiac performance studies (7,9).

RADIONUCLIDE TECHNIQUE

All studies in this laboratory have been performed using a commercially available computerized multicrystal scintillation camera (Baird-Atomic System-77) equipped with a 1½-inch parallel hole collimator. There is operator interaction with the system's 16K computer, thereby providing the opportunity for rapid processing of static and dynamic studies. An experienced operator can calculate left and right ventricular ejection fraction and left ventricular regional wall motion from a single study in less than 30 minutes. Radionuclide angiocardiograms are obtained routinely in the anterior position. For more detailed evaluation of regional wall motion, a second study is carried out in the left anterior oblique position 15 minutes later. Analysis of right ventricular performance always is obtained in the anterior position. When two sequential studies are performed (either in the same position or different positions), the first injection is made with technetium-99m sulfur colloid (10 to 15 mCi) which is cleared rapidly from the blood stream by the reticuloendothelial system. The second injection is usually made with technetium-99m pertechnetate (15 to 20 mCi); when only a single study is performed, this radiotracer is employed. Following peripheral venous injection of the radionuclide bolus, data are accumulated at 20 frames/second for approximately 25 seconds. After computer correction for the deadtime of the system and variations in inter-crystal efficiency of radiation detection, the study is replayed on the oscilloscope in serial fashion, with each image representing 20 summed 50 msec frames. Images representing the right ventricle and left ventricle are identified by study of the anatomic configuration and temporal appearance of the bolus as it passes through the central circulation. Using a magnetic pen and grid array representing the detector's 294 crystals, preliminary regions of interest are selected.

LEFT VENTRICULAR EJECTION FRACTION, EJECTION RATE, AND REGIONAL WALL MOTION

A preliminary time-activity curve is generated from the left ventricular region of interest. End-diastolic frames, identified as peaks with the highest counts, are used as starting points to sum together counts at 50-msec intervals over three to six cardiac cycles. Only cardiac cycles at the peak of the left ventricular time-activity curve are used. A series of sequential background frames then are selected directly from the left ventricular curve at a point immediately prior to the first discernible left ventricular beat (Figure 1). This background contribution represents activity overlying the heart, as well as scatter from the adjacent left atrium and lung at a time when all of the activity is in these structures. The same number of background frames as cardiac cycles chosen are summed together. This constant background is subtracted from the summed cardiac cycle, forming a high frequency, high count rate, background-corrected "representative" cycle, analogous to a relative ventricular volume curve. The left ventricular region of interest then is reconfirmed using the end-diastolic image generated from the "representative" cycle. If necessary, an updated region of interest is selected, another time-activity curve generated, and the entire process reiterated. Left ventricular ejection fraction is calculated directly from the final "representative" cycle, as counts at end-diastole, minus counts at end-systole, divided by counts at end-diastole, times 100 (6).

An excellent correlation was obtained between left ventricular ejection fraction determined by this first-pass radionuclide technique and by contrast angiography (r=0.95). The reproducibility of the technique was assessed by performing two sequential studies in the same position, separated by 20 minutes. There was no significant difference between the two studies, although individual patients did vary up to ± 3%. The feasibility of performing sequential studies in two positions also was evaluated, and an excellent correlation between left ventricular ejection fraction obtained in the anterior and left anterior oblique positions was obtained (r=0.97) (6).

Additional studies have demonstrated that appropriate selection of background is a major source of error of this technique. An experienced operator generally can identify appropriate background frames without difficulty from the contour of the left ventricular time-activity curve. However, choosing background frames too early (undersubtracting) or too late (oversubtracting) has a major effect upon the calculated ejection fraction (Figure 2). Undersubtracting background consistently results in an incorrectly low ejection fraction, while oversubtracting results in a high value. In contrast, variation in the zoning of the region of interest, as long as the proximal aorta is avoided, does not produce a consistent effect upon the calculated ejection fraction (Figure 3) (6).

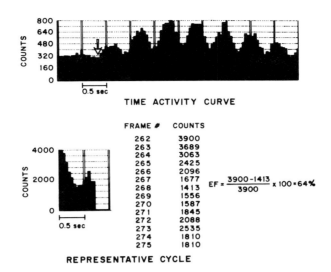

FIG. 1. Time-activity curve and "representative" cycle used to calculate left ventricular ejection fraction (EF) in a normal patient. The vertical arrow in the upper curve indicates the point of background selection. The counts for each summed 20-msec frame of the "representative" cycle are shown with the EF calculation. (Reproduced with permission from Ref. 6.)

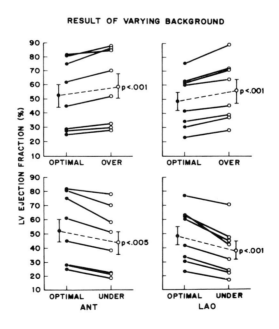

FIG. 2. Results of varying the site of background subtraction in both the anterior (ANT) and left anterior oblique (LAO) positions. Oversubtracting was produced by choosing background frames later in the left ventricular (LV) time-activity curve, while undersubtracting was produced by choosing frames earlier. Note the consistent error that is introduced by incorrectly choosing background. (Reproduced with permission from Ref. 6.)

Mean normalized left ventricular ejection rate also is obtained directly from the "representative" cycle. Using a conventional weighted least squares analysis, a straight line is fitted to the ejection phase. The slope of this line, normalized to the average number of counts during systole, represents mean ejection rate, an ejection phase index of left ventricular pump performance (normal > 2.5 sec^{-1}). This parameter was evaluated in several ways. First, left ventricular ejection rate was compared to ejection fraction obtained from contrast studies. An excellent correlation between these two indices was noted (r=0.90). Ejection rate also completely separated patients with normal and abnormal left ventricular performance (defined by contrast ejection fraction). Furthermore, there was an excellent correlation between ejection rate and the rate of circumferential fiber shortening (Vcf) determined by echocardiography (r=0.91) (10). Finally, left ventricular ejection rate was evaluated in normal subjects undergoing elective intervention studies. In the first group of five subjects, radionuclide angiocardiograms were performed at rest and following infusion of isoproterenol, a potent inotropic agent. Ejection rate increased an average of 81%, while ejection fraction rose by only 10%. These findings suggest that ejection rate may be a more sensitive indicator of pharmacologically induced changes in myocardial contractility than ejection fraction. Concomitant with the increases in ejection rate and ejection fraction, isoproterenol infusion resulted in a significant increase in heart rate. To account for any independent effects of heart rate upon this parameter, a second group of patients was studied in whom radionuclide angiocardiograms were performed at rest and following rapid atrial pacing. The elevated heart rate response, without concomitant inotropic stimulation, associated with pacing had no effect upon ejection rate, while ejection fraction fell by approximately 10% (6).

Regional wall motion analysis also is obtained from data in the "representative" cycle. Because of the high count-rate capabilities of the computerized imaging system employed, the summed end-diastolic and end-systolic images have adequate spatial resolution to permit analysis of individual analog images. These images are computer smoothed by expanding the 294 matrix points to 4704 points using a 5-point linear averaging algorithm. The outer margins of the smoothed end-diastolic image are identified visually in a standard manner based upon the color-coded isocount display. A perimeter representing the maximal end-diastolic excursion is generated by the computer. This ring then is superimposed directly upon the smoothed end-systolic image, forming a composite from which regional wall motion can be determined (Figure 4). For assessment of regional performance, sequential studies in the anterior and left anterior oblique positions are usually performed. Regional wall motion evaluated by this technique was found to agree closely with results obtained from contrast angiographic studies. In 22 patients, studied with both techniques, there was disagreement between studies in only one patient, and the site of abnormality was localized correctly by radionuclide angiocardiography in approximately 90% of abnormal segments (6).

The intrinsic variability of these parameters of left ventricular performance was assessed in multiple sequential studies in 20 stable patients with both normal and abnormal function. Individual studies were separated by at least three days. The presence or magnitude of regional wall motion abnormal-

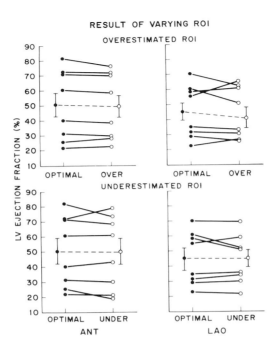

FIG. 3. Effect of varying the left ventricular (LV) region of interest (ROI) in both the anterior (ANT) and left anterior oblique (LAO) positions. No consistent effects were noted. (Reproduced with permission from Ref. 6.)

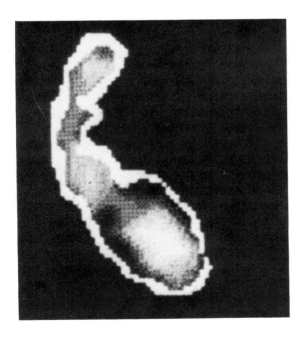 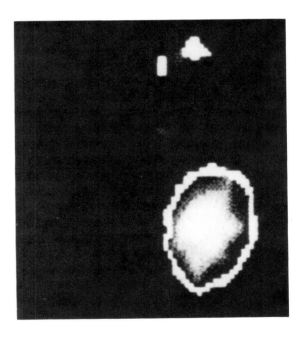

FIG. 4. Regional wall motion studies in the anterior (left) and left anterior oblique (right) positions determined from a radionuclide angiocardiogram. Computer generated end-diastolic perimeters are shown superimposed upon end-systolic images. Note the apical akinesis and anteroseptal hypokinesis.

ities did not change from study to study. For left ventricular ejection fraction, the variability averaged ($\pm$ standard deviation) 4.4$\pm$3.6%, and for left ventricular ejection rate, 0.56$\pm$0.47 sec $^{-1}$ (Figure 5). However, individual patients within that group did demonstrate interstudy variability in ejection fraction or ejection rate greater than these average values (11). These data form the basis upon which radionuclide techniques can be used to sequentially assess left ventricular performance and the effects of therapeutic interventions.

RIGHT VENTRICULAR EJECTION FRACTION

After selection of the preliminary right ventricular region of interest a right ventricular time-activity curve is generated and used to select the end-diastolic frame with the greatest number of counts and its corresponding end-systolic frame. In the anterior position, it is difficult to accurately identify the tricuspid valve plane separating the right atrium from the right ventricle. However, by subtracting the peak end-systolic image from the peak end-diastolic image, a relatively pure right ventricular region of interest can be delineated (Figure 6). In the anterior position, there is anatomic overlap between the right atrium and ventricle, resulting in a right atrial background contribution to the peak of the right ventricular time-activity curve. However, at this point, there is minimal, if any, overlap with the lungs. Thus, a reproducible background region of interest is chosen empirically as a single row of crystals adjacent to the right ventricle at the right atrial-right ventricular interface (Figure 7). The background zone is not normalized to the area of the right ventricle, because this would incorrectly assume that the entire right atrium overlaps the right ventricle. Using the computer, the right atrial curve is subtracted temporally from the right ventricular curve, yielding a high count-rate, background-corrected right ventricular time-activity curve (Figure 7) (8).

The peak end-diastolic frame is reidentified from the final curve; if it differs from the original frame chosen, the computational process is reiterated. Right ventricular ejection fraction is calculated on a beat-to-beat basis at the peak of the background-corrected time-activity curve. The final ejection fraction represents an average of the individual data (Figure 8). Beat-to-beat variation has been found to be approximately $\pm$4%.

Based upon studies in 50 clinically and hemodynamically normal subjects, right ventricular ejection fraction averaged 55%, with a normal range (mean $\pm$ 2 standard deviations) of 45 to 65%. To assess the reproducibility of this technique, seven patients were studied sequentially, separated by 20 minutes. There was no significant difference between these two studies, although individual patients varied up to $\pm$ 3%. The responsiveness of radionuclide right ventricular ejection fraction to inotropic stimulation was evaluated by performing sequential studies at rest and during isoproterenol infusion. Both heart rate and right ventricular ejection fraction increased significantly in all patients (Figure 9) (8). Because of the well-known limitations of contrast angiographic techniques for calculation of right ventricular volumes, correlative contrast

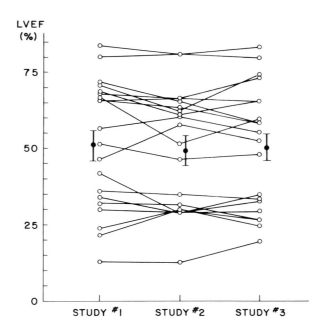

FIG. 5. Sequential studies of left ventricular ejection fraction (LVEF) separated by at least three days. There were no significant differences between studies 1, 2, and 3. Open circles represent data in individual patients. Solid circles with vertical bars represent mean ± standard deviation. (Reproduced with permission from Ref. 11.)

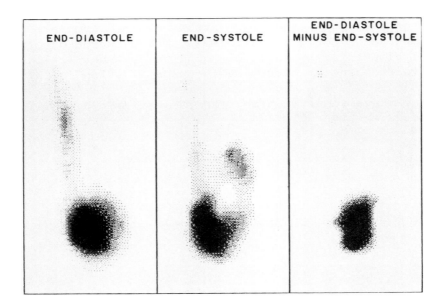

FIG. 6. Analog computer-smoothed display of peak end-diastolic and end-systolic frames used in defining the right ventricular region of interest. The end-systolic image is subtracted from the end-diastolic image to obtain the different image on the right. (Reproduced with permission from Ref. 8.)

REGIONS OF INTEREST   TIME-ACTIVITY CURVES

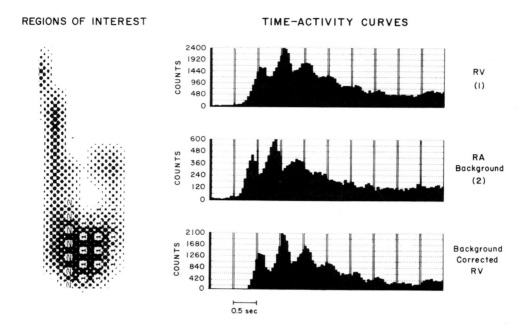

FIG. 7. Right ventricular (1) and right atrial (2) background regions of interest superimposed upon right heart image. The background-corrected right ventricular (RV) time-activity curve was obtained by subtracting the right atrial (RA) curve from the RV curve. RV ejection fraction is calculated on a beat-to-beat basis from the background-corrected RV time-activity curve. In this patient, RV ejection fraction is normal (51%). (Reproduced with permission from Ref. 8.)

ventriculographic data were not obtained as part of the validation of this radionuclide method.

The peak count rate achieved in the final background-corrected time-activity curve is critical in establishing the reliability of the angio-cardiographic data. For ejection fraction to be calculated with minimal numerical variability, high count rates are essential for adequate statistical certainty, especially in patients with abnormally low ejection fraction (Figure 8). The average peak end-diastolic count rate in either the final right ventricular time-activity curve or left ventricular "representative" cycle excedes 2000/data frame (50 msec). This provides for a statistical uncertainty of less than $\pm 3\%$.

CLINICAL APPLICATIONS AND FUTURE DIRECTIONS

First-pass radionuclide techniques have passed through the development stage and now are being applied to a variety of clinical problems and patient groups in our laboratory (8, 10, 12-18)(Table 1). One of the major clinical advantages of this approach is that data accumulation requires less than 20 seconds and thus allows rapid assessment of changing physiologic states. This also permits the study of critically ill patients who cannot remain immobilized under a scintillation camera for extended periods of time.

Recently, the first-pass radionuclide techniques described have been applied to the evaluation of global and regional left ventricular performance during supine bicycle exercise in patients with coronary artery disease (17). Patients were exercised maximally until the development of either ischemic electrocardiographic changes or rate-limiting fatigue without ischemia. In each of six normal subjects, left ventricular ejection fraction rose by at least 10% and ejection rate by at least 2.0 sec^{-1}. These increments are substantially greater than the previously established variability of the technique. Of 34 patients with documented coronary artery disease, exercise was limited by ischemia in 21 and by fatigue in 13. In the ischemic group, ejection fraction fell significantly from 65 to 56% (p<0.001). In none of the patients did ejection fraction increase beyond the variability of the technique; in eight ejection fraction remained the same, and in 13 it fell. In contrast, in the 13 patients limited by fatigue, ejection fraction increased significantly from 65 to 71% (p<0.001). Ejection fraction rose in nine patients and stayed the same in four (Figure 10). In the group of patients exercised to ischemia, mean ejection rate was unchanged. However, ejection rate increased significantly in those patients limited by fatigue (p<0.001).

Three patterns of regional wall motion responses were observed during exercise. Of the 21 patients exercised to ischemia, 12 demonstrated new regional wall motion abnormalities, two were diffusely abnormal at rest and did not change with exercise, and seven had normal wall motion at rest and during exercise. In contrast, nine of 13 patients limited by fatigue had normal wall motion both at rest and during exercise. These results demonstrate that left ventricular performance can be assessed rapidly during exercise with first-pass radionuclide angiocardiography. In addition, although exercise left ventricular function is consistently abnormal in

BACKGROUND CORRECTED RV
TIME-ACTIVITY CURVE

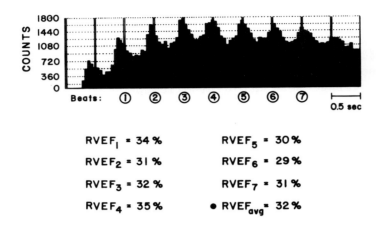

RVEF$_1$ = 34 %   RVEF$_5$ = 30 %

RVEF$_2$ = 31 %   RVEF$_6$ = 29 %

RVEF$_3$ = 32 %   RVEF$_7$ = 31 %

RVEF$_4$ = 35 %   ● RVEF$_{avg}$ = 32 %

FIG. 8. Beat-to-beat calculation of right ventricular ejection fraction
(RVEF) in a patient with cor pulmonale. RVEF is determined from counts at
end-diastole minus counts at end-systole, divided by counts at end-diastole,
times 100.

ISOPROTERENOL STUDIES

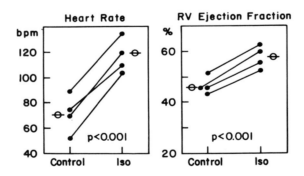

FIG. 9. Effect of isoproterenol (Iso) upon right ventricular (RV) ejection
fraction and heart rate in four subjects. Note the significant increases in
both parameters.

Table 1. Recent clinical applications of radionuclide angiocardiography at
          Yale-New Haven Hospital.

Patient Group	Type of Study	Reference
COPD	RV correlates of impaired ventilatory function	8
COPD	Effects of intravenous aminophylline upon RV and LV performance	12
Cystic Fibrosis	Detection of preclinical RV dysfunction and correlates of impaired ventilatory function	13
Thallasemia	Detection of preclinical LV dysfunction	10
ASHD	Effects of preoperative propranolol withdrawal upon LV performance	14
ASHD	Effects of institution of oral propranolol upon LV performance	15
ASHD	Serial studies of RV and LV performance in acute myocardial infarction	16
ASHD	Exercise stress intervention studies	17
Cancer	Detection of Adriamycin-induced LV dysfunction	18

COPD=chronic obstructive pulmonary disease
ASHD=atherosclerotic heart disease
RV=right ventricular
LV=left ventricular

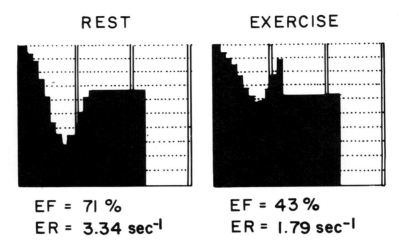

FIG. 10. "Representative" cycles determined from first-pass radionuclide angiocardiogram obtained at rest and during supine exercise in a patient with triple vessel coronary artery disease. Note the marked depression of left ventricular ejection fraction (EF) and ejection rate (ER) with exercise.

patients exercised to ischemia, the response is highly variable in patients limited by fatigue. Further studies are underway aimed at evaluating the sensitivity and specificity of these techniques.

At this time, the first-pass approach is limited in that separate injections are needed for each study. However, development of safe, short-lived, high photon-yield tracers would allow performance of multiple high count-rate studies. Recent modifications in the multicrystal camera now allow accumulation of up to 400,000 counts/second at a rate of 50 frames/second. These advances will permit calculation of minimal and maximal ejection rates during the ejection phase, development of diastolic phase indices representative of ventricular compliance, and evaluation of regional ejection fractions. Future directions also will include improved super-imposition of the end-diastolic and end-systolic images used to evaluate regional wall motion; such modifications would take into account the known intrinsic rotation and movement of the heart during contraction.

In conclusion, the efficacy of first-pass radionuclide angiocardiography for combined assessment of right and left ventricular performance has been established. Based upon the current data, noninvasive evaluation of cardiac performance with these techniques will become an increasingly valuable clinical approach.

ACKNOWLEDGEMENTS

The major contributions of Dr. Robert C. Marshall are gratefully acknowledged, as are the assistance of Ms. Coletta Sawyer and Ms. Linda Pytlick.

REFERENCES

1. Van Dyke D, Anger HO, Sullivan RW, et al: Cardiac evaluation from radioisotope dynamics. J Nucl Med 13: 585, 1972.

2. Weber PM, dos Remedios LV, Jasko IA: Quantitative radioisotopic angiocardiography. J Nucl Med 13: 815, 1972.

3. Schelbert HR, Verba JW, Johnson AD, et al: Nontraumatic determination of left ventricular ejection fraction by radionuclide angiocardiography. Circulation 51: 902, 1975.

4. Steele P, Kirch D, Matthews M, et al: Measurement of left heart ejection fraction and end-diastolic volume by a computerized, scintigraphic technique using a wedged pulmonary arterial catheter. Amer J Cardiol 34: 179, 1974.

5. Steele P, Van Dyke D, Trow RS, et al: Simple and safe bedside method for serial measurement of left ventricular ejection fraction, cardiac output, and pulmonary blood volume. Br Heart J 36: 122, 1974.

6. Marshall RC, Berger HJ, Costin JC, et al: Assessment of cardiac performance with quantitative radionuclide angiocardiography: Sequential left ventricular ejection fraction, normalized left ventricular ejection rate, and regional wall motion. Circulation 56: 820, 1977.

7. Budinger TF, Rollo FD: Physics and instrumentation. Prog Cardiovasc Dis 20: 19, 1977.

8. Berger HJ, Matthay R, Loke J, et al: Assessment of cardiac performance with quantitative radionuclide angiocardiography: Right ventricular ejection fraction with reference to findings in chronic obstructive pulmonary disease. Amer J Cardiol, In press 1978.

9. Grenier RP, Bender MA, Jones RH: A computerized multi-crystal scintillation gamma camera. In, Instrumentation in Nuclear Medicine, vol 2 (Hine GJ, Sorenson JA, eds), New York, Academic Press, 1974.

10. Hellenbrand W, Berger HJ, O'Brien R, et al: Left ventricular performance in Thalassemia: Combined noninvasive radionuclide and echocardiographic assessment. Circulation 56: Suppl III, III-49, 1977 (abst).

11. Marshall RC, Berger HJ, Reduto LA, et al: Variability in sequential measures of left ventricular performance assessed by radionuclide angiocardiography. Amer J Cardiol, In press 1978.

12. Berger HJ, Matthay RA, Gottschalk A, et al: Effects of aminophylline on right and left ventricular performance in chronic obstructive pulmonary disease: Assessment by quantitative radionuclide angiocardiography. Clin Res 25: 208, 1977 (abst).

13. Matthay RA, Berger HJ, Loke J, et al: Right and left ventricular performance in cystic fibrosis: Assessment by noninvasive radionuclide angiocardiography. Chest 72: 407, 1977 (abst).

14. Reduto LA, Berger HJ, Marshall RC, et al: Serial radionuclide assessment of left ventricular performance during propranolol withdrawal prior to aortocoronary bypass surgery. Circulation 56: Supp III, III-195, 1977 (abst).

15. Marshall RC, Berger HJ, Reduto LA, et al: Effect of oral propranolol upon left ventricular performance in coronary artery disease: Noninvasive assessment by sequential radionuclide angiocardiography. Circulation 56: Suppl III, III-32, 1977 (abst).

16. Reduto LA, Berger HJ, Cohen L, et al: Sequential radionuclide assessment of left and right ventricular performance following acute myocardial infarction. Circulation 56: Suppl III, III-65, 1977 (abst).

17. Borkowski H, Berger HJ, Langou R, et al: Rapid assessment of left ventricular performance during exercise-induced myocardial ischemia: First pass radionuclide technique. Circulation 56: Suppl III, III-198, 1977 (abst).

18. Alexander J, Dainiak N, Duffy T, et al: Prospective noninvasive assessment of adriamycin-induced cardiac dysfunction using serial radionuclide angiocardiography. Clin Res, In press 1978 (abst).

THE USE OF THE NUCLEAR STETHOSCOPE
FOR TEMPORAL IMAGING OF LEFT VENTRICULAR FUNCTION

Henry N. Wagner, Jr.

The Johns Hopkins Medical Institutions
Division of Nuclear Medicine
Baltimore, Maryland 21205

Diseases of the left ventricle can be divided into three pathophysiological groups: (1) volume overload, as in aortic or mitral insufficiency or left-to-right shunts; (2) pressure overload, as in systemic-hypertension or aortic stenosis; and (3) diseased myocardium, as in coronary artery disease or idiopathic myocarditis. Differentiation of the relative importance of each of three factors in a given patient can often be made by looking at changes in the volume of blood within the left ventricle as a function of time. For example, in patients with valvular heart disease, by looking at ejection fraction we can see how well left ventricular performance has adapted to the mechanical load placed on it by the valvular lesion. A low ejection fraction indicates excessive dilatation or concommitant myocardial disease. Other evidence of myocardial failure is prolongation of the pre-ejection period of the ventricle and shortening of left ventricular ejection time. In patients with hypertension or aortic stenosis, we have observed that diastolic filling is slower and more prolonged than normal, even before myocardial failure has occurred, as indicated by a low ejection fraction. We have also been able to assess the responsiveness of the ventricle to stimulation by drugs or to various maneuvers, such as Valsalva, or exercise.

All of these data can be obtained from a left ventricular function curve, provided temporal resolution is adequate and the changes in recorded radioactivity levels correspond to changes in the volume of blood within the left ventricle.

Certain clinical problems in cardiology require a high degree of spatial resolution for their solution while others require a high degree of temporal resolution. For example, to detect a small area of the myocardium being supplied by a stenosed coronary artery requires maximum spatial resolution, even if this must be achieved at the cost of some temporal resolution. In such cases, it is at times best to view two high spatial resolution images, one end-systolic and the other end-diastolic. On the other hand, if we are concerned with overall or global ventricular function, we may prefer an image of the temporal changes that occur within the entire ventricle during the cardiac cycle. Such temporal images, displaying changes over a period of time as short as 10 milliseconds may be preferable to spatial images. It depends on whether we are concerned primarily with temporal or spatial relationships.

In choosing the proper technical solution according to the nature of the problem, we constantly face the problem of photon limitation. To increase either spatial or temporal resolution or both, we need to increase the number of available photons, but we are always limited by radiation dose. Therefore, we must make choices.

Which are we to emphasize in a given situation, spatial or temporal resolution? It depends on the nature of the problem. Two of the most fundamental adaptive mechanisms of the left ventricle in the face of disease are hypertrophy and/or dilatation. We might assume that high resolution spatial images would be best for detection of these states, but in preliminary studies, we have evidence to suggest that temporal imaging of the rate of filling of the heart may be an even more sensitive index of hypertrophy than direct visualization of wall thickness in nuclear images.

We have observed the effects of an increased mechanical load against which the heart must pump blood, as in aortic stenosis or systemic arterial hypertension, by high resolution temporal rather than spatial images. We have observed prolongation of the pre-ejection period (PEP), a decrease in the rate or duration of left ventricular emptying and a decrease in the rate of ventricular filling; to do so, we believe that a temporal resolution of 10 milliseconds is required.

What about dilatation? It is possible that a non-imaging detector might be adequate for detection of cardiac dilatation, in a manner analogous to the use of a non-imaging detector in the detection of hyperthyroidism, but an imaging device would seem clearly preferable.

What about after compensatory mechanisms have failed? In such cases, temporal patterns have again shown promise of being ideal for detection of the abnormality, in evaluating the response to treatment, and in monitoring the course of the disease.

The pulsatile nature of ventricular function makes it possible to achieve both high spatial and temporal resolution, but only at the cost of time. For example, to obtain a ventricular function curve with a spatial matrix size of 32 x 32 picture elements over the region of the left ventricle with a temporal resolution of 64 intervals per cardiac cycle requires approximately 10 minutes. With a device designed specifically to provide temporal patterns with spatial resolution limited to the field of view of the detector, as in the nuclear stethoscope, we can observe beat by beat changes in ventricular function. This capability is ideally suited for perturbation studies, such as graded exercise or Valsalva maneuver, or to detect the immediate effect of drugs, or to monitor sudden changes in ventricular function in the coronary care unit or even on the operating table (Fig. 1).

Of course, the validity of these temporal imaging techniques remains to be demonstrated, but initial results have been encouraging. In the case of nuclear imaging techniques, comparison with contrast ventriculography has indicated that contrast ventriculography and nuclear methods correlate surprisingly well, particularly in view of the differences under which the two types of studies are performed: contrast angiography requires a cardiac catheter to be in place and the administration of contrast media that has a striking hemodynamic effect, and is much more traumatic than the nuclear study. The temporal imaging methods, such as the use of the nuclear stethoscope, have been less extensively compared, but results have been encouraging.

In a series of patients in whom the results with the nuclear stethoscope were compared to scintillation camera-computer studies, the correlation coefficient was between 0.80 and 0.86, the latter figure being observed in the last 21 comparisons as the physicians became more experience in the use of the nuclear stethoscope (Fig. 2).

The most frequently asked question about the nuclear stethoscope is about positioning. How can we be sure we are viewing the left ventricle properly?

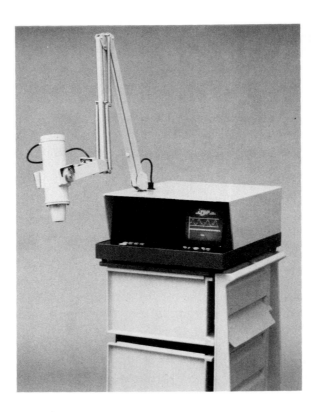

FIG. 1. The latest version of the nuclear stethoscope.

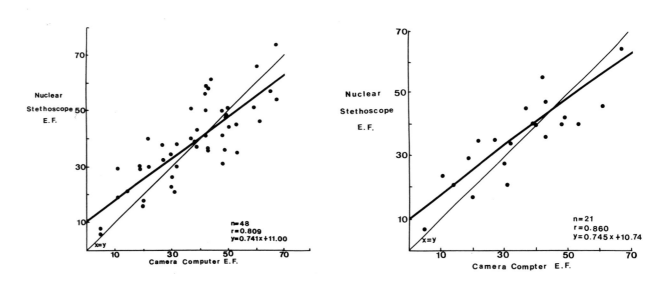

FIG. 2. (Left) Correlation between measurements of ejection fraction with
the nuclear stethoscope and with the Anger camera. Each value is the average
of three observations made independently by three observers. These are comparisons in the first 48 patients. (Right) The same correlation in the subsequent 21 patients. We believe that the better correlation is the result
of experience in the use of the nuclear stethoscope.

There are two characteristics of the nuclear stethoscope that make it possible to position the detector properly: (1) the real-time display of the ventricular function curve (Fig. 3) permits the physician to look at the curve and then calculate ejection fraction as he moves the detector from one position to another over the chest wall. He does so until certain easily defined criteria have been met. These are: (a) end-diastolic activity must be approximately twice background; and (b) stroke volume must be maximum. The first criterion eliminates the possibility that only the edge of the ventricle is being viewed. The second criterion ensures that the entire left ventricle, but not the right ventricle, left atrium or aorta are in the field of view.

After the detector has been positioned over the ventricle, the time-activity curve is then obtained by integrating the measurements over 1 to 4 minutes (approximately 70 to 280 beats) dividing the R-R interval into at least 100 points (Fig. 4). Two representative cardiac cycles are viewed to facilitate examination of the diastolic phase of the cardiac cycle, as well as the systolic.

(2) In studying the effects of exercise or other perturbations, such as drugs, the detector is kept in the same position relative to the patient by means of an arm that holds the detector in position. If the heart remains within the field of view of the detector throughout the study and background activity does not change unpredictably, then positional effects are minimized.

Initial experience with the nuclear stethoscope has suggested that positioning problems are less than with the Laennec stethoscope or echocardiogram. With all three devices, the immediate availability of the results permits correct positioning by trial and error.

In addition to the problem of whether to opt for spatial or temporal imaging, we are faced with the question of whether to emphasize the first transit of the tracer through the heart or to wait until the tracer has distributed itself throughout the vascular compartment. Even when the decision has been made to emphasize equilibrium studies, the first transit of the tracer is usually monitored to provide information regarding transit times. Such information is useful in evaluation of transpulmonary transit times, pulmonary blood volume, and cardiac output.

A question arises with respect to whether direct measurement of right and/or left ventricular function (i.e., ventricular time-activity curves) can be obtained satisfactorily in first transit studies, or whether the tracer should be allowed to equilibrate in the vascular compartment prior to obtaining the curves.

Among the questions involved in this decision are:

(1) Are the activity levels high enough to permit adequate spatial and temporal resolution in first transit studies?
(2) In achieving statistically adequate counting rates, can problems of limited temporal responsiveness (dead time) be solved?
(3) Are the greater number of views possible with the equilibrium method a compelling advantage?

Valsalva

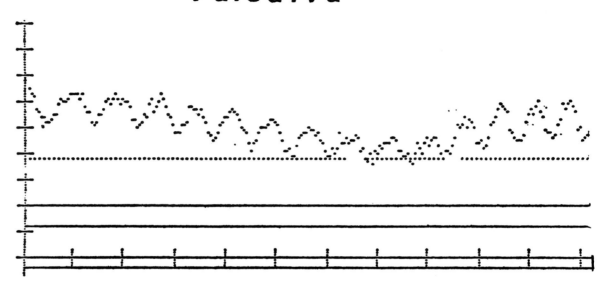

FIG. 3. Temporal image of the radioactivity level within the left ventricle as observed in real time with the nuclear stethoscope. The effect of Valsalva maneuver is apparent.

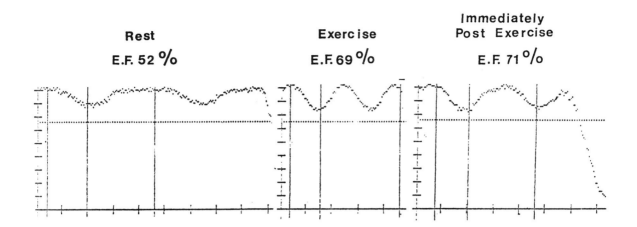

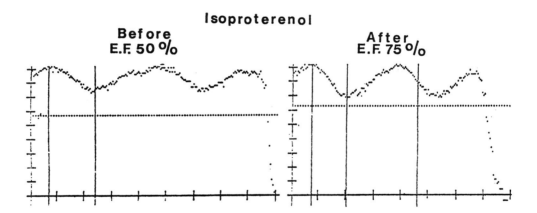

FIG. 4. (Top) Temporal images of the left ventricular time-activity curves. The effect of exercise in shortening the R-R interval and increasing ejection fraction is apparent. (Bottom) The effect of inhalation of isoproterenol on ventricular function curve. The shortening of the R-R interval and the increase in ejection fraction is apparent.

(4) How many views are required in the first transit studies?
(5) Is the problem of background activity significantly less with first pass methods?
(6) Are positioning problems greater for some systems more than others?

Even if the final answer to these questions were known, neither time nor space would permit their adequate consideration here.

Instead, I shall describe our initial results related to some of these problems.

BACKGROUND

In extensive studies with the equilibrium method, background levels averaged approximately 50% of end-diastolic activity. It is clear that considerable variability results from where background is selected. If the left atrium, pulmonary arteries, or aorta are within the field of view, background will be high and ejection fraction correspondingly low. We have found and reported elsewhere that reproducibility among three independent observers is good if careful attention is paid to avoiding the chambers and vessels that fill during systole. To date, we have found the region above the spleen, below the pulmonary arteries and immediately adjacent to the lateral wall of the left ventricle gave consistently best results.

An important question is whether background changes during the particular perturbation, such as exercise, under study. Initial results in our laboratory are still uncertain. In some patients during exercise, background activity has not changed significantly, while in others it has. Further study is being made of this important point, particularly in the case of monitoring studies with the nuclear stethoscope.

TEMPORAL RESOLUTION

We have found that dividing the cardiac cycle into 64 points is adequate for measurement of pre-ejection period and rates of emptying and filling of the left ventricle. Temporal resolution is best in the case of the nuclear stethoscope, and probably not completely satisfactory if the cardiac cycle is divided into only 16 time intervals. Of course, if we are satisfied with only ejection fraction, a temporal resolution of 0.20 or 0.25 second might be adequate.

SPATIAL RESOLUTION

We have observed that considerable improvement in image quality occurs when a 64 x 64 image cell matrix covers the region of the left ventricle. Thirty-two x 32 cell images seem much less satisfactory. Interpolation of the image cells up to 256 x 256 or 512 x 512 image cells is helpful, but is not as good as recording the original data in at least a 64 x 64 cell matrix.

DEAD TIME PROBLEMS

Clearly one of the major advantages of the 294-crystal imaging system, known as the System 77, is its excellent temporal responsiveness, probably

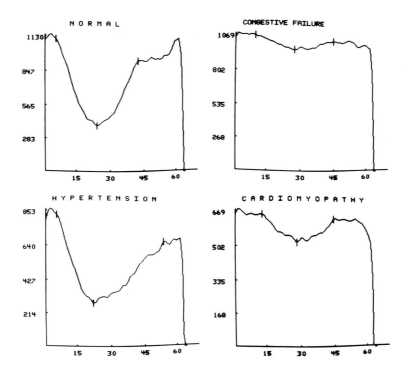

FIG. 5. Characteristic patterns of ventricular function curves in the diseases indicated.

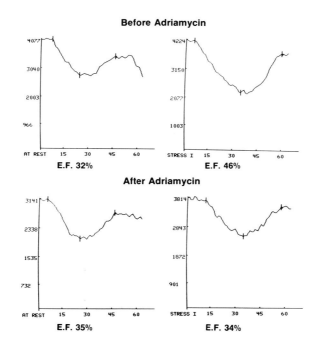

FIG. 6. Ventricular function curves before and during exercise in a patient who received adriamycin for treatment of lymphoma. After adriamycin treatment, the ejection fraction did not rise with exercise.

ten times better than with the Anger systems. The high counting rates and small dead times make it possible to perform right and left ventricular wall motion and global functional measurements using only the first transit data. At present we are comparing first transit studies with this system and equilibrium studies with the Anger camera, in the same patients on the same day. Subsequently we plan to study whether dead time problems with the Anger camera are an insurmountable problem for accurate measurement of ventricular function using only first transit data.

CLINICAL RESULTS

Characteristic left ventricular function curves have been obtained in patients with heart failure and in patients with pressure overload, not in failure (Fig. 5).

Changes in ventricular function can be monitored effectively with either the scintillation camera or nuclear stethoscope. A major advantage of the latter is that the data are immediately available. Examples are shown in Figure 6.   It is likely that both systems will be used more and more, each for its own particular purpose.

REFERENCES

1. Wagner HN, Jr., Wake R, Nickoloff E, et al: The Nuclear Stethoscope: A Simple Device for Generation of Left Ventricular Volume Curves. Amer. J. Cardiol. 38: 747-750, 1976.

2. Bacharach SL, Green MV, Borer JS, et al: A Real-Time System for Multi-Image Gated Cardiac Studies. J. Nucl. Med. 18: 79-84, 1977.

3. Lotter MG, Douglass KH, Knowles LG, Nickoloff EL, Wagner HN Jr: A Technique for the Evaluation of Global and Regional Ventricular Function. Proceedings of 7th Symposium on Sharing of Computer Programs, National Technical Information Service, U.S. Dept. of Commerce, Springfield, Virginia 2216, CONF-770101.

4. Wagner HN Jr: The Nuclear Stethoscope: A Bedside Device for Continuous Monitoring of Ventricular Performance. Circulation 52, Supplement II, October, 1975.

5. Ashburn WL, Kostuk WJ, Karliner JS, Petesen KL, Sobel BE: Ventricular Volume and Ejection Fraction Estimation by Radio-Nuclide Angiography. Semin. Nucl. Med. 3: 165-176, 1973.

6. Bacharach SL, Green MV, Borer JS, Ostrow HG, Redwood DR, Johnston GS: ECG-Gated Scintillation Probe Measurement of Left Ventricular Function. J. Nucl. Med. 18: 1176-1183, 1977.

7. Qureshi S, Wagner HN Jr, Nickoloff EL, et al: Evaluation of Left Ventricular Function in Normal Persons and Patients with Heart Disease. J. Nucl. Med. 19: 135, 1978.

A SIMULATED HEART MODEL USING COMPUTER IMAGE ANALYSIS

FOR VALIDATING CARDIOVASCULAR NUCLEAR MEDICINE PARAMETERS

Robert R. Hurst, Ph.D., Department of Physics,
University of Missouri-Columbia and
K. William Logan, Ph.D., Richard A. Holmes, M.D.,
Harry S. Truman Veterans' Administration Hospital,
Columbia, Missouri, 65201

ABSTRACT

Computer quantization of various cardiovascular nuclear medicine procedures have generally been applied without an accurate validation of the many parameters employed to obtain the data. In spite of this, the clinical application of these techniques continues to grow with many of the initial questions and problems that tend to degrade the results still unanswered or unsolved. To better understand these problems and generate quantitative solutions we have constructed a versatile heart simulator, (Dynamic Universal Heart Model Y'all)(DUHMY) to measure such parameters as ejection fraction accuracy, chamber volumes, effects of variable background, effects of absorption and scattering, detection of wall motion, and the effect of different collimation on image resolution. The results of the measurements are given and discussed.

INTRODUCTION

Figure 1 shows DUHMY which is constructed of heat-tempered glass and is essentially the volume of a large human heart (525 ml) with two balloon chambers driven by a variable speed Harvard respiratory pump. The model differs from the one developed by the Johns Hopkins group because of its six variably adjustable bleeder valves that allow the two chambers (balloons of different size and shape) to dilate and contract at variable rates, phases, and volumes. Easily readable graduated cylinders hold the perfusing liquids. The heart is inserted into a large opened-top glass cylinder simulating the thoracic cavity.

Radionuclide imaging measurements of DUHMY were obtained for various combinations of volume and count rate; linearity was achieved until rather large ventricular volume, and high count rate (greater than 5×10^5 cpm) were reached using an Ohio Nuclear 120 System Mobile Camera. Similarly ejection fractions with different background configurations were measured. A trigger pulse was obtained using a micro switch mounted so that it was triggered with each pump motor revolution. This gated the Digital Equipment Corporation PDP-11/40 analyzer with the x-y recording of data being accomplished using two analog-to-digital converters. Regions of interest were drawn using the joy stick mode and total counts were obtained for the "end diastolic" and "end systolic" configurations. All measurements were obtained using the same camera/computer system used regularly in our laboratory for clinical cardiac studies.

The static volume and multiple gated "heart" dynamic studies of DUHMY were acquired in 32 x 32 matrix mode and processed to provide quantitative results of the above effects. The ventricular time activity curves, gross and net count rates for ventricles, the observed laboratory versus computer calculated ejection fractions as functions of total count rate and background, are then compared to examine the accuracy and validity of similar clinical patient radionuclide studies.

EJECTION FRACTIONS

The computer was gated by a trigger pulse shaped similar to the R-wave pulse obtained with an ECG. Counts were then recorded in 47 frames of 30 milliseconds each. The time activity curves were similar to those shown in Figures 2 and 3. Background corrections were made if necessary and the regions of interest were drawn using the joy stick at peak maximum (end diastolic) and the curve minimum (end systolic). This was done by three independent observers with little or no deviation in the values obtained. The ejection fraction data are presented in Table 1.

BACKGROUND ABSORPTION AND SCATTERING EFFECTS

The effects of scattering, absorption and background activity were studied with no water around DUHMY, water but no activity, and with activity and water in the surrounding cylindrical cavity. The background was subtracted by taking regions of interest near the balloons; the results are

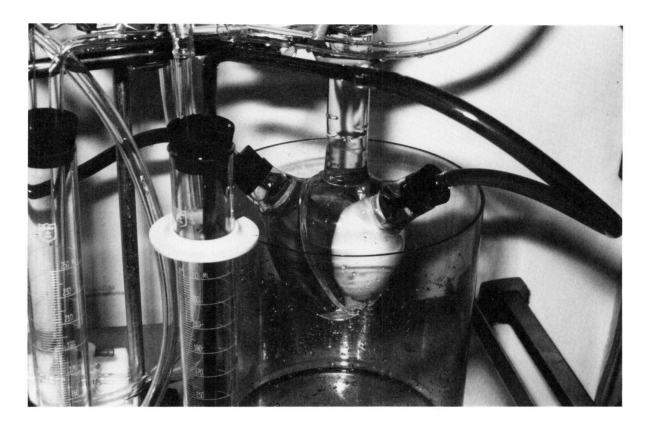

FIG. 1. DUHMY Heart Model.

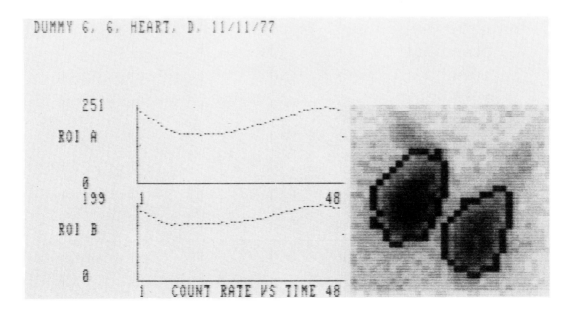

FIG. 2. Ventricular time-activity curves for region A (left upper) and region B (right lower) balloons.

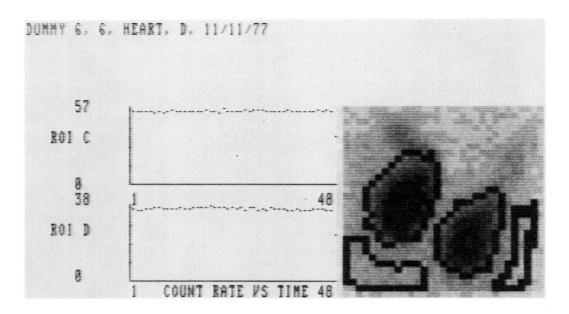

FIG. 3. Time-activity curves for background regions.

TABLE 1.   COMPARISON OF EJECTION FRACTION VALUES
           OBTAINED USING OHIO NUCLEAR 120 SYSTEM

Identification	Using Graduated Cylinder Data	Using Computer Analysis
DUMMY 26	0.603	0.618
DUMMY 19	0.565	0.554
DUMMY 20	0.565	0.547
DUMMY 21	0.565	0.547
DUMMY 22	0.565	0.548
DUHMY 2	0.472	0.496
DUHMY 3	0.362	0.388
DUMMY 33	0.300	0.316
DUMMY 34	0.300	0.313
DUHMY 1	0.264	0.265

essentially in agreement with DUHMY alone. Figure 4 illustrates the linearity of the system with no background activity. Figure 5 gives the results with activity in DUHMY and the cylindrical cavity. Only after a balloon contained more than 110 milliliters did absorption become apparent with the data points falling increasingly below the straight line in the figure. Observe that after an appropriate subtraction for background, the results are very similar to those shown in Figure 4, the slopes being nearly identical.

WALL MOTION

The lower limits of detectable wall motion were investigated using a Tc-99m solution injected into one of the balloons which was filled to different static volumes and imaged with the camera. At each different static volume light from a slide projector located three meters away was used to cast a shadow of the inflated balloon on a piece of graph paper positioned two centimeters behind the balloon, the paper being taped to the collimator on the mobile camera. The images were traced with pencil with an estimated error of no greater than 0.5 mm. (see Figure 6). Each different static volume was collected in 64 x 64 and 128 x 128 matrices for later display and analysis with the computer. In order to further validate quantitative comparisons, a four-inch square hole was cut in a piece of lead which covered the face of the camera (without collimator). A Tc-99m sample was positioned two meters away from the camera and the image from the four-inch opening was recorded in the two matrix sizes.

Different methods were used to enhance the simulated travel of the wall as represented by the images. Matrix subtraction provided reasonable definition of the location of the balloon wall motion (Figure 7); however, matrix division of the larger image by the smaller often appeared to yield a more definitive difference (see Figure 8). Examination of the wall motion data provided the following information: Using 128 x 128 collection mode gave a "full width at half max" of the enhanced adjacent image of 2.5 mm as best minimum; using 64 x 64 collection mode gave 5.0 mm as the best minimum.

DIFFERENT COLLIMATION

Three different straight-bore collimators were used: an all-purpose, a high-sensitivity, and a high-resolution. As expected, the count rate was much lower with the high-resolution and highest with the high-sensitivity. However the lower limit of resolution for the wall motion appears to depend more on the size of the image matrix than the camera collimation for the collimators and other parameters used in this study. We are making a new series of measurements to determine more quantitatively the effect of camera collimation on wall motion detection.

CONCLUSIONS

DUHMY is providing a method of testing and validating current and new techniques for imaging and quantitatively analyzing dynamic cardiac function and motion. Absorption and scattering of 140 Kev photons have been shown to have relatively little effect on accurate ejection fraction determination.

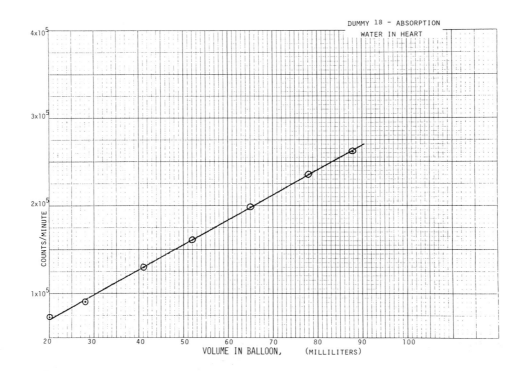

FIG. 4. Count rate vs. balloon volume in ml with no background.

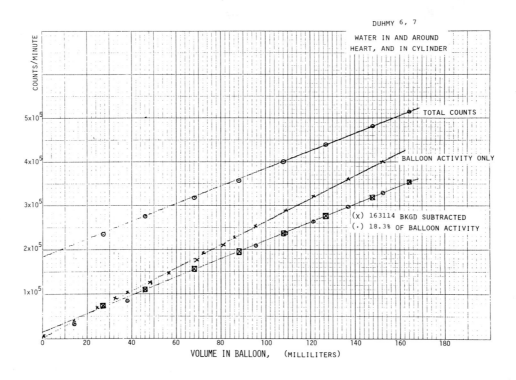

FIG. 5. Count rate vs. balloon volume in ml with background activity; same data with indicated background subtracted.

The validity of background subtraction has been examined, indicating that
even with the high background levels found in clinical studies, background
subtraction can achieve accurate results. DUHMY also has shown that
extremely low ejection fractions (less than .30) can be determined accurately.

The study of wall motion with DUHMY suggests that surpisingly small
(2-3 mm) dimensions of wall motion can be detected. The limits of wall
motion detecton and quantification have been shown to depend on image matrix
size in addition to resolution limits due to collimation.

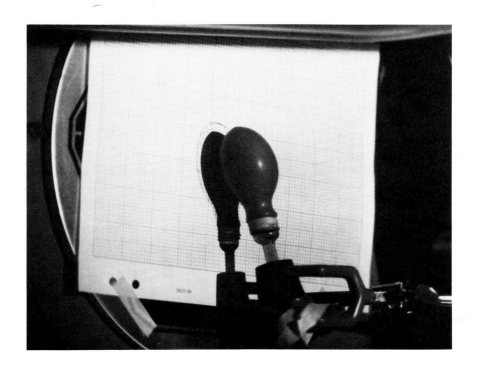

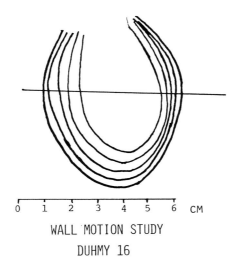

WALL MOTION STUDY

DUHMY 16

FIG. 6. (Top) Illustration of method used to outline balloon image for wall
motion studies. (Bottom) Typical curves obtained using method shown at
top.

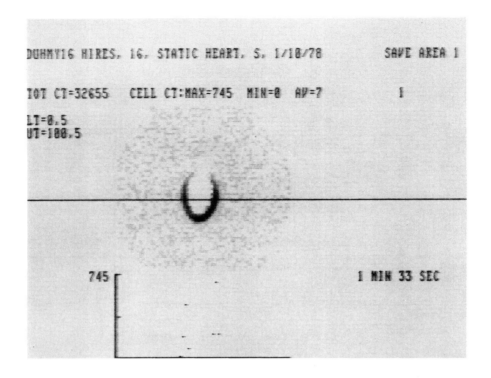

FIG. 7. Result of matrix subtraction of adjacent images obtained using high-resolution collimator in 64 x 64 storage mode.

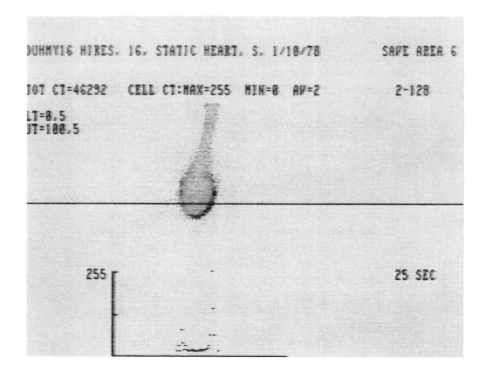

FIG. 8. Result of matrix division of adjacent images obtained using high-resolution collimator in 128 x 128 storage mode.

CYCLICALLY GATED CARDIAC STUDIES
WITH R-R INTERVAL-DEPENDENT WINDOW WIDTHS

George B. Bell, Ben W. Spade,
and Paul O. Scheibe

Biomedical Research Department,
Analytical Development Associates Corporation
Sunnyvale, California

Malcolm R. Powell

Suite 908
350 Parnassus Avenue
San Francisco, California 94117

ABSTRACT

Changes in R-R interval alter the phasic relationship between cyclically gated images and cardiac events when fixed image window times are used. A computer program has been developed which monitors the R-R interval on a beat-by-beat basis during the examination, predicts each next R-R interval from a running weighted average, excludes bad beats, and normalizes the images after the study to compensate for any timing errors during accumulation. The program has been tested in rest and stress studies.

INTRODUCTION

The calculation of ejection fraction and other clinical parameters from cyclically gated cardiac data depends on a constant phasic relationship between the images of the cycle and critical cardiac events. Most cyclically gated techniques acquire images using fixed image window durations determined from R-R intervals measured just prior to image acquisition (1, 2, 3). Changes in R-R interval, however, alter the image-event relationship if image windows of fixed duration are used. This is particularly true in stress studies.

We have developed a computer program for monitoring R-R intervals during the examination and for making real-time adjustments to image window duration to compensate for heart rate changes.

METHOD

In our technique, as in those of other investigators (1, 2, 3), each cardiac cycle is divided into n segments. The temporal resolution is proportional to n, where n may be 16 for a 64 x 64 x 8 matrix or 32 for a 32 x 32 x 8 matrix in our system.* Additionally, the n segments can be distributed over any desired percentage of the R-R interval from 20 to 100 percent starting with each R-wave (Figure 1). This allows the operator to increase temporal resolution during systole by imaging only the first part of the cardiac cycle. During cyclic data acquisition, images representing each segment of the cardiac cycle are stored in computer memory and displayed for the operator in a cine mode. At any time during acquisition, the operator may elect to erase image memory without otherwise interrupting the study. This allows the operator to reposition the patient or eliminate images acquired before the patient reached equilibrium stress conditions. At the conclusion of data acquisition, images are transferred to disc for storage and recall purposes (Figure 1).

The system monitors the R-R interval on a beat-by-beat basis prior to and during image collection. A weighted average R-R interval is calculated after each heart beat to predict the next R-R interval using the formula shown below:

$$_pT_n = (_pT_{n-1} \times w) + (_aT_{n-1} \times (1-w))$$

where $_pT_n$ = next predicted R-R interval

$_pT_{n-1}$ = last predicted R-R interval

$_aT_{n-1}$ = last actual R-R interval

w = weighting factor (0.7)

---

*The method discussed in this paper was programmed on an LSI-11 microprocessor with 56 Kbytes of program memory and 64 Kbytes of video memory.

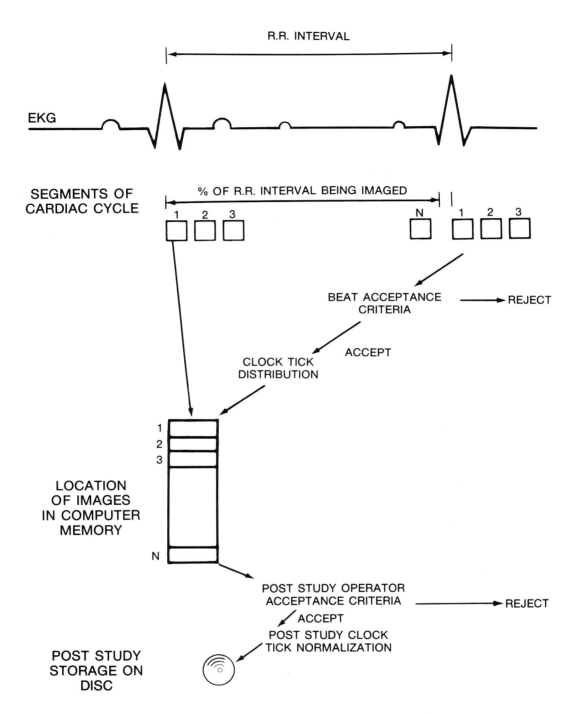

FIG. 1. Cyclically gated imaging technique.

Beat Acceptance Criteria. At the time each R-wave is detected, the hardware system clock is reset (Figure 2). In the time between reset and the first integer clock tick (0.01 sec for a 100 Khz clock), the system calculates the "next predicted R-R interval" from the above equation. Each actual R-R interval is compared to the predicted interval, and data collection starts when five consecutive R-R intervals are within ± 20% of their predicted values (Table 1).

When an R-R interval is detected that differs by more than ± 20% from its predicted value, the next five heart beats will be rejected. However, most or all of the images from the bad cycle will already have been stored by the time the bad R-wave is detected. This is indicated by parentheses in Table 1. A tally of these bad cycles is maintained and will be discussed subsequently.

The system will not calculate a "next predicted R-R interval" immediately after an interruption to preclude biasing the running weighted average by one ectopic beat. Next predictions will be calculated from the next two R-R intervals regardless of their duration in case a major change in heart rate has occurred. The third interval following a bad beat will be tested to see if it falls within ± 20% of the new predicted interval as a test of the prediction. Data collection will be restarted on the sixth beat following an interruption if the last three beats prior to the sixth beat fall within ± 20% of their predicted values.

Clock Tick Distribution. Each segment of a cycle is started and stopped on the basis of a specific clock tick number but the clock tick numbers for any segment may vary from beat to beat. The first segment of any cycle starts on the first clock tick after the clock is reset (Figure 2). The ending clock tick for that segment and the starting and ending ticks for every other segment are calculated from the formula:

$$t_i = \frac{(S_i)\,(P)\,(_pt_n)}{100n} + fr$$

where t_i = ending clock tick number for the ith segment, and starting clock tick number for the (i^{th} + 1) segment

S_i = the ith segment number of the cardiac cycle ($1 \leq i \leq n$)

P = percent of cardiac cycle to be imaged (operator specified)

$_pt_n$ = number of clock ticks for "next predicted R-R interval"

n = number of segments per cycle (16 or 32)

and fr = a rounding factor of 1, 1 + 1/n, 1 + 2/n, 1 + 3/n, ..., or 2.

t_i is an integer formed by truncating the fractional part of the right-hand expression in the above equation. The rounding factor, fr, is constant for all segments in a cycle but progresses through permissible

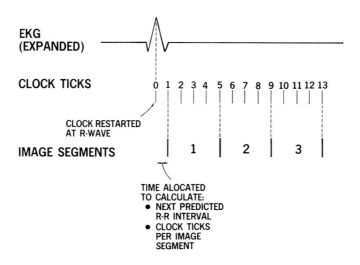

FIG. 2. Image segment timing technique.

TABLE 1.   BEAT ACCEPTANCE/REJECTION CRITERIA

Preceding Four R-R Intervals*	Penultimate R-R Interval*	Last R-R Interval		Next R-R Interval
IN	IN	IN	ACCEPT	ACCEPT
IN	IN	OUT	(ACCEPT)	REJECT
EITHER	OUT	OUT	REJECT	REJECT
EITHER	OUT	IN	(REJECT)	REJECT

*Note: "IN", "OUT", and "EITHER" refer to an R-R interval being "WITHIN" or "OUTSIDE" $\pm$ 20% of its predicted interval.

values to distribute integer truncation errors which might accumulate in some segment if the heart rate remains constant. The effect of the rounding algorithm is illustrated in the appendix.

Post-Study Operator Acceptance. As indicated in the above discussion of the beat acceptance criteria, some or all images associated with a bad beat will be stored. At the conclusion of data acquisition but before storage on disc occurs (Figure 1), the program reports the total number of cycles and the number of bad cycles acquired. The operator may then decide to accept the study (store on disc) or erase and redo the study.

Post-Study Clock Tick Normalization. A tally of the accumulative number of clock ticks per segment is maintained during each study. If the operator elects to accept a study, the system will normalize the image data to correct for differences in the accumulative number of clock ticks in each segment. These differences might occur because of clock tick truncation errors or cycles incompletely imaged because of premature R-waves. The normalization will be performed by multiplying every pixel of each segment by an appropriate factor to normalize image window duration with respect to the segment with the smallest number of accumulative clock ticks. If the difference in clock ticks in the longest and shortest segment is more than 15% of the longest, the study will not be normalized and the operator will be given an opportunity to redo the study. This might occur if the total number of cycles acquired is too small to allow the rounding factor to be effective.

Verification Techniques. To test the clock tick distribution and post-study normalization algorithms, a flood field was imaged while the system was gated by a normal subject's EKG. Parameters for the study were selected so 16 images were obtained for each cycle, but the percentage used in separate studies included 50%, 90%, 95% and 100%. The counts in each frame were ascertained and the mean and standard deviation calculated.

To test the ability of the system to follow changes in heart rate, a subject with normal sinus rhythm was imaged while seated upright on a bicycle ergonometer. Parameters for the study were selected so the 16 images were distributed over 90% of the R-R interval following each R-wave event. Data were accumulated while the subject's heart rate increased from resting to stress levels.

RESULTS

Results of the clock tick distribution and post-study normalization test where a flood field was imaged over 90% of a normal subject's R-R interval are shown in Figure 3. The counts in each frame are within three standard deviations of the mean which would be expected in 99.7% of the frames due to Poisson counting statistics.

In data not presented in this paper, it was discovered that if 95% or 100% of the R-R interval was imaged, one or more frames contained counts in excess of three standard deviations from the mean. It was also discovered that the algorithm did not work well if a very small number of cycles (e.g., 15) were imaged. In such cases, the system reported it was unable to normalize the frames and the operator was given an option to redo the study.

In the test of the system's ability to follow changes in heart rate from rest to stress levels, a cyclic sequence of 16-segment images was observed in real time on the display screen of the system. As the patient exercised, the rate at which images were displayed on the screen increased. Occasional interruptions in the display were observed and were attributed to gating events outside the 20% window.

An activity cycle curve from the left ventricle for a subject at rest is shown in Figure 4.

DISCUSSION

Green reported the first clinical use of a multiple-image cyclic gated technique and observed a trail-off (decrease in counts) in the left ventricular activity-cycle histogram at late diastole due to small changes in the R-R interval (1). Bacharach observed the same phenomenon and proposed a scheme for eliminating the trail-off of data by merging two activity-cycle curves (4). Both curves started at the R-wave but one curve was formed by progressing forward from the R-wave and the other progressing backward. The merged curve consisted of the first two-thirds of the forward curve, and the late-diastolic one-third of the reverse curve. A user-selected beat-length window was also employed.

Bacharach's method has the advantage of defining very late diastolic events, such as atrial contraction, and does compensate for random variations in R-R interval associated with a steady heart rate. His technique requires either real-time analysis of buffered data or list mode storage and post-study processing.

Our objective was to develop a system that would be convenient for the operator to use, exclude data when the heart rate changes abruptly, and compensate for a gradual drift in heart rate expected in stress studies.

The beat acceptance criteria in our method, although using an arbitrarily determined 20% window, provides immunity for the system against a series of bad gating events which might occur in a temporary arrythmia, electrical lead readjustment, muscle noise, or an EKG base-line shift.

The problem of eliminating data from a single ectopic beat has not been solved by our method (Table 1) although the operator is provided with a tally of the total number of beats acquired and the number of bad beats included in the tally. This provides the clinician with an indication of the validity of a study, or a warning that a study should be repeated or interpreted with caution. Although it was not attempted in this study, data from a single bad beat could be eliminated by using 2 or 3 buffer areas in memory; data from each beat could be acquired in a buffer and a decision made after each R-wave to exclude data, or to transfer it to a memory storage area. More than one area would be needed in order to give the system time to transfer data to the storage area. Such a scheme was not attempted in our present system because

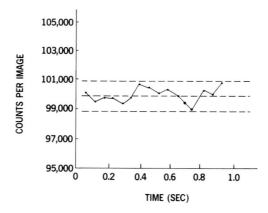

FIG. 3. Counts in each frame of a flood field study imaged while the system was gated over 90% of a normal subject's R-R interval.

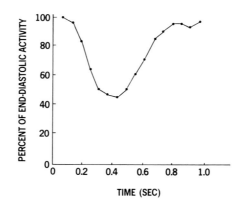

FIG. 4. Activity cycle curve from a resting patient imaged over 90% of the R-R interval.

it would not be possible to include 16 segments in a 64 x 64 matrix and still have room in memory for buffers.

Updating the predicted R-R interval after each beat compensates for gradual changes in the average heart rate in rest or stress studies. The weighting factor, although arbitrarily chosen, makes the system responsive to change, while insuring that the system is most strongly influenced by the running average heart rate.

The method we have developed does not attempt to adjust to continuously varying R-R intervals which occur, for example, in atrial fibrillation. In that disease state, each beat would not be predictable from previous beats. Although not attempted, a system which would successfully image a patient with atrial fibrillation might be developed using the buffer scheme suggested above. Only beats meeting certain criteria would be stored.

The results of testing clock tick distribution and post-study normalization indicate the algorithm successfully distributed truncation errors when 90% or less of the R-R interval was imaged and a sufficient number of beats accumulated. Counts in excess of three standard deviations from the mean occurred when imaging 95% and 100% of the R-R interval. For that reason, we have subsequently been imaging over 90% or less of the R-R interval on our system. Excessive count variation while imaging more than 90% of the R-R interval might have been due to premature R-waves occurring during the acquisition of an image segment. When an R-wave occurs while an image is being acquired, the system immediately stops acquiring data. Since this won't necessarily coincide with a clock tick, the counts accumulated from the last clock tick to the premature R-wave contribute to the segment being imaged but the corresponding time is not accounted for. Even though this time is less than 10 msec, the effect of premature beats in the same segment would be accumulative.

The rest and stress test conducted on the subject with normal sinus rhythm was not a typical clinical protocol for a stress study. Data were accumulated continually from rest to stress in order to observe data accumulation over widely varying heart rates. Normally, data would not be accumulated over such extremes in heart rate because the systolic phase of the cardiac cycle occupies an increasingly greater portion of the R-R interval because the diastolic phase is shortened as the heart rate increases.

A clinical protocol for stress studies would be to start imaging as the patient begins exercise to verify patient positioning. At the point where the desired level of stress is obtained, data in memory would be erased. A control key is provided so the operator can erase memory without otherwise interrupting data acquisition. This permits the rapid transition to data acquisition once the desired level of stress is reached.

APPENDIX

The rounding factor is composed of two parts, a constant 1.0 to allow for the fact that timing starts at clock tick 1, and a fraction to distribute truncation errors through the segments without accumulation of errors in any segment. For example, a given R-R interval may result in a desired

acquisition time of 3.3 clock ticks per segment. The calculated starting
and ending times for the first four segments would be as follows:

Segment Number	Start Tick (Ideal)	Stop Tick (Ideal)	Interval	Total After 16 Beats
1	1	4.3	3.3	52.8
2	4.3	7.6	3.3	52.8
3	7.6	10.9	3.3	52.8
4	10.9	14.2	3.3	52.8
.				
.				

Since we can't start or stop at fractional ticks, this table would actually
be as follows:

Segment Number	Start Tick (Actual)	Stop Tick (Actual)	Interval	Total After 16 Beats
1	1	4	3	48
2	4	7	3	48
3	7	10	3	48
4	10	14	4	64
.				
.				

After several beats with the same R-R time, we have an accumulated error of
33% in one frame. To avoid this problem, the rounding factor changes after
each beat and the above table would be replaced by one of n tables (where n
is the number of segments per beat). The following table is composed of the
first segment entry in each of the 16 tables (for a 16-segment study).

Segment #1

	Rounding Factor	Start Tick	Stop Tick	Interval
1	1.0	1	4	3
2	1.0625	1	4	3
3	1.1250	1	4	3
4	1.1875	1	4	3
5	1.2500	1	4	3
6	1.3125	1	4	3
7	1.3750	1	4	3
8	1.4375	1	4	3
9	1.5000	1	4	3
10	1.5625	1	4	3
11	1.6250	1	4	3
12	1.6875	1	4	3
13	1.7500	1	5	4
14	1.8125	1	5	4
15	1.8750	1	5	4
16	1.9375	1	5	4
				52

The tables for each of the other segments have the same numbers, in a different order for each table, so after 16 beats with the same R-R interval, the collection times for each segment will be the same. Note also that 52 clock ticks were accumulated after 16 beats in the above example and that corresponds very closely to the ideal number of clock ticks, 52.8, which would be obtained if fractional ticks were possible.

REFERENCES

1. Green MV, Ostrow HG, Douglas MA, et al: "High temporal resolution ECG-gated scintigraphic angiocardiography." *J Nucl Med* 16:95-98, 1975

2. Bacharach SL, Green MV, Gorer JS, et al: "A real-time system for multi-image gated cardiac studies." *J Nucl Med* 18:79-84, 1977

3. Folland ED, Hamilton GW, Larsen SM, et al: "The radionuclide ejection fraction: a comparison of three radionuclide techniques with contrast angiography." *J Nucl Med* 18:1159-1166, 1977

4. Bacharach SL, Green MV, Borer JS, et al: "ECG-gated scintillation probe measurement of left ventricular function." *J Nucl Med* 18:1176-1183, 1977

FRAME-RATE REQUIREMENTS FOR RECORDING TIME-ACTIVITY CURVES BY RADIONUCLIDE ANGIOCARDIOGRAPHY

Glen W. Hamilton, M. D.;
David L. Williams, Ph.D.; and James H. Caldwell, M. D.

Veterans Administration Hospital
Nuclear Medicine and Cardiovascular Disease Sections
Seattle, Washington 98108

ABSTRACT

The optimum frame rate for recording the left ventricular time-activity curve at rest and during exercise has not been determined, although it is generally appreciated that high frame rates result in "statistical noise," due to inadequate counts, and that low frame rates will not produce an accurate activity curve.

We have examined high fidelity time-volume curves obtained by cine-radiography at rest and during progressive exercise. The signal frequency spectra of the volume curves showed that greater than 95% of the frequency content of the curves is below 7 Hz. Based on the fundamental sampling theorem, these curves should be accurately reconstructed by data collected at greater than twice this frequency or 14 samples per second.

An additional problem is the long sample period used with radionuclide techniques to provide adequate counts in the recorded data. Sampling over this finite time span causes a slight but definite decrease in amplitude of the time-activity curve, even when the sampling rate is greater than twice the maximum frequency component of this function.

Both these principles were confirmed by sampling actual rest-exercise volume curves at progressively slower frame rates and longer sample periods. The results demonstrate that there is a slight decrease in the calculated ejection fraction as frame rate is decreased from 120 to 15-20 frames per second due to the long sample period. When the frame rate is lower than 15 frames per second, gross errors in ejection fraction are observed. These are due to sampling at less than twice the highest frequency component of the left ventricular volume curve, a phenomena known as aliasing.

Based on these observations, a frame rate of about 25 frames per second seems to be optimum to maintain both accuracy in the recorded data and adequate counting statistics.

INTRODUCTION

Radionuclide angiocardiography following a radiotracer injection attempts to capture data related to volume, size, and shape of the cardiac chambers as a function of time. These data may be generated during the first transit of the tracer or during the blood-pool equilibrium phase, and are recorded in either the form of serial images or time-activity curves. Since the important physiologic information is contained in the temporal variations, it is important to understand the principles of accurately sampling and recording these data. This paper reviews the sampling theory relevant to recording left ventricular dynamic function, and presents a model demonstrating the effect of frame rate on the ejection fraction determined from radionuclide data-recording techniques.

SAMPLING: TERMINOLOGY AND REVIEW

The procedure by which a continuous signal (analog signal) is transformed into a discrete time-digitized signal (digital signal) is called sampling and is characterized by two concepts: sample rate and sample period. The sampling rate, or frequency, is the number of samples collected per unit time. It is equal to $1/T$, where T is the time between samples and is expressed in frames per second (FPS). The sample period, or aperture , is the length of time over which each sample is collected. The signal frequency spectrum refers to the distribution of sinusoidal frequency components which can mathematically represent a waveform. It is obtained by "decomposition" of the primary waveform into an ensemble of sinusoidal waveform components by Fourier analysis. The fundamental sampling theorem states that an arbitrary signal must be sampled at a rate at least twice the highest frequency component in its spectrum to preserve the harmonic content in the sampled data (1,2).

Bove, et al. have studied frame rate requirements for contrast biplane cineangiocardiography at rest (3,4). Using a sampling rate of 270 FPS with a sample period of 0.00075 seconds, they generated continuous left ventricular volume curves. The frequency spectrum calculated by Fourier analysis demonstrated that more than 95% of the frequency content was below 8 Hz. Based on this finding, they predicted that a frame rate of 16 FPS would be adequate and confirmed experimentally that the left ventricular volume curve could be accurately regenerated from samples taken at this frame rate.

SAMPLING FOR RADIONUCLIDE STUDIES

Radionuclide studies present special sampling problems, due to the statistics of decay and the limited number of counts available for recording. For example, if one samples radionuclide data using 60 FPS and a sample period of 0.004 seconds (as is commonly used for contrast cineangiography), too few counts will be obtained with resultant large statistical errors. For this reason, the sample period for nuclear studies must be increased greatly and is commonly set at the reciprocal of the frame rate (i.e., at a frame rate of 25 FPS, the sample period is 1/25 second) so that all data are collected.

The effect of sample period on the frequency content of the recorded data is shown in Fig. 1. Note that there is virtually no decrease in relative response up to 25 Hz when the sample period is short, e.g., 0.004 seconds, as is commonly used for contrast cineangiography. Likewise, with sample periods of 0.01 and 0.02 seconds (corresponding to frame rates of 100 and 50 FPS for nuclear medicine studies), there is little decrease in relative response up to frequencies known to contain the majority of the left ventricular frequency components (8-10 Hz). However, when the sample period is longer (illustrated by the 0.04 and 0.10 second sample periods used for radionuclide studies with frame rates of 25 and 10 FPS), the relative response of the sampling system is diminished at frequencies known to be contained in the left ventricular time-volume curve (i.e., 0-8 Hz). Thus, when the sample period is quite short, as in contrast angiography, the accuracy of the recorded data is dictated almost totally by the sampling rate selected. When sample periods are relatively long, such as used for radionuclide studies, the accuracy is dependent upon both sample rate and sample period.

Based on these concepts, we previously studied cineangiographic time-volume curves from four resting patients and determined the decrease in calculated ejection fraction (EF) that would occur with progressively slower frame rates and lengthening sample periods (5). With the sample period equal to the reciprocal of the frame rate, there was less than a 1% decrease in EF at 25 FPS and less than 2% decrease at 16 FPS when the heart rate was less than 80 per minute. When the heart rate was 105 per minute, there was a 2% decrease in EF as the frame rate was slowed to 25 FPS. We concluded that resting studies of EF could be accurately performed with a frame rate of 25 FPS and that higher frame rates increased statistical noise without enhancing accuracy.

This paper extends these observations to left ventricular time-volume curves obtained at higher heart rates during exercise, to define the frame rate requirements for recording rest-exercise radionuclide measurements of EF. Additionally, the volume curves presented were determined from surgically implanted metallic clips and are essentially noise free, making possible a more accurate calculation of the signal frequency spectrum than previously possible (3,4).

METHODS

Eight left ventricular time-volume curves, obtained from two patients who had surgically implanted metallic clips on the ventricle, were selected for study. The two patients selected demonstrated the largest change in heart rate and/or ejection fraction among a group of nine patients studied to assess postoperative left ventricular function (6). For each patient, ventricular time-volume curves were obtained at rest and at 300, 600, and 900 KPM exercise levels. At each level, cineangiography was performed at a sampling rate of 60 FPS and a sample period of 0.004 seconds, with volume calculated from changes in the spatial relationships between the clips (6).

The signal frequency spectrum was determined from each curve by Fourier analysis. Each curve was then interpolated to 120 points per second and

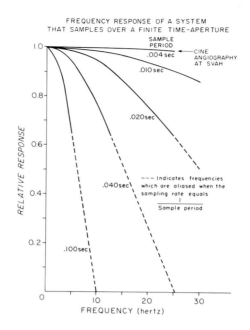

FIG. 1. The relationship between relative system response and sample
period. With a sample period of 0.004 seconds, the relative system response
remains nearly 1.0 up to 25 Hz. With sample periods commonly used with
radionuclide studies, e.g., 0.10 and 0.04 seconds corresponding to frame
rates of 10 and 25 FPS, the relative system response is reduced at frequencies which compose the left ventricular volume curve (1-8 Hz). The dotted
portions of the curve denote regions in which the sampling frequency is
less than twice the sampled frequency and where aliasing will occur.

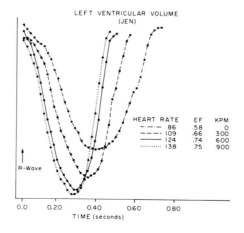

FIG. 2. Left ventricular volume curves obtained by 60 FPS cineradiography
of surgically implanted metal clips. Curves were obtained at rest and
three levels of exercise on a bicycle ergometer. During exercise, there is
an increase in both ejection fraction and heart rate.

progressively reduced to 60, 40, 30, 24, ...6 samples per second by averaging 2, 3, 4, 5, ...20 successive points on the curve, starting at the R-wave. The effect of averaging is exactly analogous to collection of the data with radionuclide gating techniques, at progressively slower frame rates with a sample period equal to 1/(frame rate). From each curve generated, end-diastolic volume (EDV), end-systolic volume (ESV), and ejection fraction (EF) were determined and plotted as a function of frame rate.

RESULTS

The eight time-volume curves studied are shown in Figs. 2 and 3. The patient shown in Fig. 2 demonstrates an increase in EF (0.58 to 0.75), heart rate (86 to 138), and the rate of ventricular ejection and filling during exercise. The systolic ejection period (R-wave to end-systole) decreases from 0.40 to 0.28 seconds. The patient illustrated in Fig. 3 shows little change in ejection fraction or the rate of ejection, in spite of an increase in heart rate from 89 to 167. The systolic ejection period decreases from 0.32 to 0.22 seconds.

The signal frequency spectra of the rest-exercise left ventricular volume curves shown in Fig. 2 are presented in Fig. 4. It is apparent that the majority of the frequency content is below 3-4 Hz. For the curve with the lowest heart rate and EF, 95% of the frequency content is below 4.3 Hz; for the curve with maximal frequency content during exercise, 95% was below 6.8 Hz. Ninety-seven percent of the frequency content, even at the maximal EF and heart rate, was below 12 Hz.

The effect of frame rate on EDV, ESV, and EF is shown in Fig. 5. As frame rate is reduced, there is a slight decrease in EDV and EF, and a slight increase in ESV down to a frame rate of 15-20 FPS. Below this level, a marked decrease in EDV and EF, and a marked increase in ESV is noted. The other seven curves were qualitatively identical, although at slower heart rates the changes were less pronounced and the sharp decrease in EDV and EF occurred at a lower frame rate.

Fig. 6 illustrates the changes in EF as frame rate was reduced; three curves are shown for each patient (lowest, moderate, and highest heart rate). Each curve shows a similar pattern with a minor decrease in EF down to a sampling rate of about 20 FPS and then a pronounced fall at about 10-15 FPS. As would be expected, the fall in EF is least at low heart rates (86 and 67) and greatest with high heart rates (138 and 167). Note also that the frame rate at which the EF begins to decrease markedly is higher with higher heart rates. The magnitude of the gradual decrease in EF noted above 20 FPS is small; the EF decreasing from an average of 0.522 at 120 FPS to 0.500 at 20 FPS.

DISCUSSION

The data presented here provide a logical basis for the selection of an appropriate frame rate for recording left ventricular time-activity curves if the parameters to be measured are known. Simple inspection of the volume

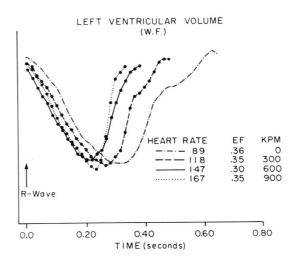

FIG. 3. Left ventricular volume curves obtained from a postsurgical patient
as in Fig. 2. During exercise, there is a marked increase in heart rate
with little change in ejection fraction.

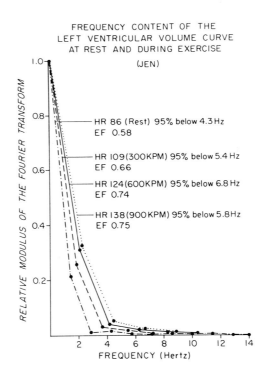

FIG. 4. Signal frequency spectra obtained by Fourier analysis of the ventricular curves shown in Fig. 2. A clear shift toward higher frequencies
is noted in the curves recorded during exercise. Even in the curve with
the highest frequency content, 95% of the frequency spectrum was below
7.0 Hz.

curves in Figs. 2 and 3 shows that a sampling rate of 60 FPS with a short sample period is quite adequate for recording a high-fidelity curve even at high heart rates. It is also apparent that some portions of the left ventricular volume curve, for instance, the pre-ejection period or the phase between rapid and slow ventricular filling, would require more than 60 FPS for accurate delineation. However, for most purposes, the information desired is end-diastolic and end-systolic volume or activity for calculation of EF. The current study is directed specifically at the selection of an optimum frame rate for determining the EF.

The definition of a minimum frame rate to record the EF accurately at varying heart rates and ejection fractions is not academic. It takes three times as long to record a curve at 60 FPS than it does at 20 FPS if the same statistical accuracy is maintained. With the current emphasis on measuring transient changes in EF (over seconds to minutes) following pharmacologic or physiologic interventions, it is important that each measurement of EF be performed rapidly.

To determine the optimum frame rate, we have examined rest-exercise ventricular volume curves from the standpoint of sampling theory and by a model identical to the radionuclide data-collection technique, where the sample period is inversely proportional to the frame rate. Fourier transform analysis of the signal frequency spectra reveals that 95% of the frequency content is below 7 Hz, even when ejection fraction and heart rate are high. The fundamental sampling theorem predicts that the curve should be accurately reconstructed from data collected at any sampling rate greater than twice this frequency (7 Hz) if the sample period is short. However, at a sampling rate of 14 Hz, there will be some loss of amplitude, due to the long sample aperture as shown in Fig. 1. This model, which shows ejection fraction decrease as frame rate is decreased when the sample period equals 1/(frame rate), behaves as one would anticipate from sampling theory; below a sampling rate of 14 FPS, there are gross errors in the calculated EF, due to aliasing in the frequency domain. At frame rates above 14 Hz, there are rather slight decreases in EF, as frame rate is reduced, due to loss of high frequency response caused by the long sample period.

Based on these data, a frame rate of about 25 FPS appears to be optimal. This rate will cause a slight underestimation of EF, due to a relatively long sample period, but is high enough to avoid large aliasing errors induced by sampling at less than twice the maximum frequency contained in the volume or activity curves. Further, this rate provides relatively good counting statistics. As an alternative, the data could be recorded at a much higher frame rate with a shorter sample period and post-processed with a low-pass digital filter to minimize statistical variations. Depending on filter characteristics, the final curve would have nearly the same frequency content as a curve recorded at a sampling rate twice the filter cutoff level. The latter technique should, however, minimize the slight decrease in EF, due to a relatively long sample period, and merits further investigation.

We had anticipated that a major increase in heart rate, such as seen with exercise, would cause a major shift in the signal frequency spectrum toward higher frequencies. In fact, this shift was definite but minimal (Fig. 4). Likewise, in the frame rate model, the frame rate effects were only slightly

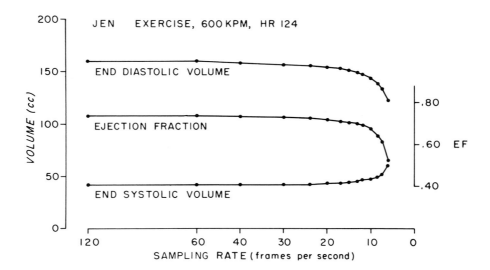

FIG. 5. Relationship of EDV, ESV, and EF to sampling rate as frame rate
was decreased with a sample period equal to 1/(frame rate). Very slight
changes in EDV, ESV, and EF are noted as frame rate was decreased to
15-20 FPS. Below this level, EDV and EF decreased rapidly and ESV increased markedly. The gradual decrease above 15 FPS is due to increasing
sample period. The rapid fall in EF below 15 FPS is due to sampling at
a rate less than twice the highest frequency present in the data.

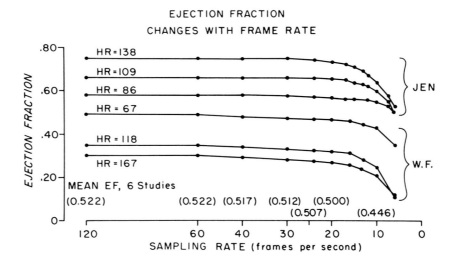

FIG. 6. The relationship of EF to frame rate at varying levels of exercise.
The EF curves are from the two patients shown in Figs. 2 and 3. In both patients, when the heart rate is low, the EF decrease is slight, down to 10
FPS and then falls rapidly. At higher heart rates, the rapid fall in EF
occurs at a higher frame rate.

greater at high heart rates. This is likely because the major change with
an increased heart rate is shortening of the diastolic filling time with a
lesser decrease in the systolic ejection period.

ACKNOWLEDGEMENTS

This study was supported in part by the Veterans Administration and
NHLI Grant #1R01-HL-18805-01. We acknowledge the typing assistance of
Mrs. Katharine Jelsing; and the technical assistance of our medical illustra-
tor, Ms. Joy Godfrey, and photographer, Mr. Clinton Kolyer.

REFERENCES

1. Shannon CE: Communication in the presence of noise. Proc IRE 37:
    10-21, 1949.

2. Landau HJ: Sampling, data transmission, and the Nyquist rate.
    Proc IEEE 55: 1701-1706, 1967.

3. Bove AA, Ziskin MC, Freeman E, et al: Selection of optimum cine-
    radiographic frame rate, relation to accuracy of cardiac measurements.
    Invest Radiol 5: 329-335, 1970.

4. Freeman E, Ziskin MC, Bove AA, et al: Cineradiographic frame rate
    selection for left ventricular volumetry. Radiology 96: 587-591,
    1970.

5. Hamilton GW, Williams DL, Gould KL: Selection of appropriate frame
    rates for radionuclide angiography. J Nucl Med 17: 556, 1976 (abst).

6. Vine DL, Dodge HT, Frimer MJ, et al: Quantitative measurement of left
    ventricular volumes in man from radio-opaque epicardial markers.
    Circulation 54: 391-399, 1976.

OPTIMUM COUNTING INTERVALS IN RADIONUCLIDE CARDIAC STUDIES

Kevin W. Bowyer, George Konstantinow, Jr.,
Stephen K. Rerych, and Robert H. Jones*

Duke University Medical Center
Department of Surgery
Nuclear Cardiology Laboratory
Durham, North Carolina 27710

*Howard Hughes Medical Investigator
This work supported in part by National Institutes of Health
Grants HL 20677 and HL 17670

ABSTRACT

This study examines the relationship between counting interval and heart rate in first-pass radionuclide studies. Using a Baird-Atomic System Seventy-Seven multi-crystal gamma camera, seventeen radionuclide angiocardiograms were acquired at 10-msec counting intervals. Subject heart rates (HR) at time of study ranged from 63 to 217. Summation of consecutive data frames provided data equivalent to counting intervals at 10-msec increments from 20 to 100 msec. Using derived left ventricular volume curves, the optimal counting interval (OCI) was determined for each study. The OCI in msec as a function of heart rate was determined to be OCI = 37 - .11 X HR. Reliable images of the left ventricle required a 40-msec counting interval at slow heart rates and a 20-msec interval at rapid heart rates.

INTRODUCTION

Radionuclide angiocardiograms provide rapid noninvasive assessment of many important parameters of cardiac function. Data recorded during initial transit of tracer through the central circulation has been used to assess valvular insufficiency (1), determine chamber-to-chamber transit times (2) and detect and quantitate intracardiac shunts (3,4). Changes in left ventricular counts during cardiac contraction permit assessment of left ventricular function (5). Comparison of ventricular function at rest and during exercise appears to be of great diagnostic value in patients with ischemic heart disease (6,7). Highly sensitive gamma cameras are essential for accurate measurement of left ventricular function from a single transit of tracer. Moreover, the count accumulation interval can influence the left ventricular volume curve and ejection fraction measurement, particularly at the high heart rate associated with exercise studies. Thus, the optimal counting interval (OCI) should be sufficiently long to permit statistical accuracy of data but sufficiently short to reflect the full range of ventricular volume change during cardiac contraction. The purpose of this investigation was to define the OCI for radionuclide angiocardiogram data obtained with a total counting rate of 300,000 counts per second obtained from the initial transit of a radionuclide bolus through the heart.

METHODS

A Baird-Atomic System Seventy-Seven multi-crystal gamma camera in our laboratory was recently modified with a high frame rate feature which permits acquisition of dynamic data at 10-msec counting intervals (8,9). Using this instrument, seventeen radionuclide angiocardiograms were obtained. Ten studies were recorded during rest and seven studies were recorded with subjects exercising in the erect position on a Fitron bicycle ergometer. Heart rates during the seventeen studies ranged fairly evenly from a low of 63 to a high of 217 beats per minute. The 15-mCi dose of technetium-99m pertechnetate was selected because two separate administrations of this amount of tracer are commonly used in our laboratory for rest and exercise studies performed sequentially. A one-inch collimator was used which permits a maximum counting rate of 380,000 counts per second with administration of 30 mCi of technetium-99m pertechnetate. The total counting rate achieved from 15 mCi averaged 300,000 counts per second. The counting rate achieved was lower than would be expected because of a 2-msec period of data loss between each 10-msec accumulation interval which represents the time necessary for transfer of data from buffer memory to disc.

Initial data processing corrected for instrument dead time and detector nonuniformity (10). In subjects studied with more than one injection, residual background radioactivity was determined and subtracted from the subsequent study. Data recorded at 10 msec was summed to provide data at 10-msec increments from 20 to 100 msec. The left ventricular evaluation program of the Baird-Atomic System Seventy-Seven Volume II software was used to construct a left ventricular volume curve, left ventricular image, and ejection fraction at each of the ten counting intervals for each of the seventeen patients. Details of the software used for left ventricular evaluation have been previously reported (11). The program combines counts recorded over the left ventricle during multiple consecutive cardiac contractions into a single representative or average cardiac cycle which has greater statistical accuracy than data recorded during

individual heart beats. A left ventricular volume curve and ejection
fraction are obtained from this representative cardiac cycle. In addition,
static and cine images of contraction permit assessment of left ventricular
wall motion. Supraimposition of volume curves at each of the ten counting
intervals for each of the seventeen patients studied permitted construction
of a volume curve which appeared to most accurately reflect left ventricular
contraction. The mean of the squared differences between the ideal
curve and each of the ten observed left ventricular volume curves was
determined using the IBM 370/165 computer. The OCI was defined to be
the counting interval with the minimum mean squared difference from the
ideal volume curve.

Static and dynamic images of left ventricular contraction during
the representative cardiac cycle were inspected at each counting interval.
A subjective determination of the accumulation interval which first
provided an image with sufficient anatomic definition to permit left
ventricular volume determination was tabulated. Determination of the
optimal imaging interval was made by two observers without knowledge of
the optimal counting interval determined from the left ventricular
volume curve.

Patients were divided into three groups based upon a heart rate
less than 100 (6 patients), heart rate of 100 to 150 (6 patients), and
heart rate greater than 150 (5 patients). The mean percent error in
ejection fraction was determined for each group at each counting interval.

RESULTS

Measurements of ejection fraction at each of the count intervals
are recorded in Table 1. These data demonstrate the counting interval
to influence the ejection fraction less in patients with slow heart
rates than in patients studied with high heart rates. Ventricular
volume curves in a patient with a heart rate at 63 show statistical
fluctuation and temporal distortion is particularly apparent in data
recorded at 10 msec (Fig. 1). Timing of end-systole and end-diastole is
influenced by the statistical quality of data and is different for each
of the three curves. Although the actual ejection fraction of the 10-
msec curve is .80, appropriate selection of end-diastole would result in
an ejection fraction of .62 which differs only slightly from the ejection
fraction of .60 at 50 msec. Both the 50-and 100-msec curves provide
similar assessment of left ventricular function in this patient. Left
ventricular volume curves in a patient with a heart rate of 217 show
obvious distortion in the 100-msec curve due to the relatively long
counting interval (Fig. 2). Although the 10-msec curve obviously provides
the closest approximation of the biologic function, the 50-msec curve
provides a fair representation of left ventricular volume changes even
at this rapid heart rate. Images constructed at varying counting intervals
in a patient with a heart rate of 66 demonstrate the reliability of the
end-diastolic parameter to increase with longer counting intervals
(Fig. 3). Although the 30-msec image could be used for left ventricular
volume determination, images at longer counting intervals would prove
more satisfactory. Images obtained in a patient with a heart rate of
184 show great statistical fluctuation in the 10-msec image (Fig. 4).
The 30-msec image could be used for volume determination. The optimal
counting interval for imaging the left heart in this patient appears to
be 50 msec and a less accurate evaluation of wall motion is apparent at
longer counting intervals.

TABLE 1. EJECTION FRACTION OBTAINED AT DIFFERENT COUNTING INTERVALS

	COUNTING INTERVALS (msec)									
PATIENT HEART RATE	100	90	80	70	60	50	40	30	20	10
63	.49	.52	.52	.55	.54	.54	.55	.55	.61	.78
66	.73	.74	.76	.74	.73	.74	.79	.74	.82	.83
77	.39	.43	.43	.42	.44	.44	.43	.54	.58	.61
94	.62	.61	.67	.63	.64	.64	.66	.69	.73	.80
98	.80	.81	.80	.78	.79	.79	.81	.85	.85	.90
98	.60	.60	.62	.64	.64	.64	.71	.69	.76	.92
100	.51	.52	.53	.53	.54	.52	.58	.58	.63	.65
101	.65	.65	.65	.67	.70	.68	.69	.71	.72	.78
110	.66	.66	.65	.66	.66	.69	.68	.72	.71	.71
120	.63	.66	.66	.72	.69	.73	.74	.75	.79	.79
133	.60	.62	.63	.66	.67	.66	.70	.71	.72	.80
150	.67	.69	.72	.72	.75	.79	.80	.83	.84	.77
171	.54	.57	.59	.65	.64	.67	.69	.68	.72	.73
184	.52	.60	.61	.64	.68	.65	.70	.68	.70	.78
200	.68	.73	.74	.76	.78	.81	.83	.84	.89	.89
203	.44	.46	.51	.55	.59	.62	.63	.65	.68	.70
217	.62	.60	.67	.66	.71	.76	.75	.78	.81	.85

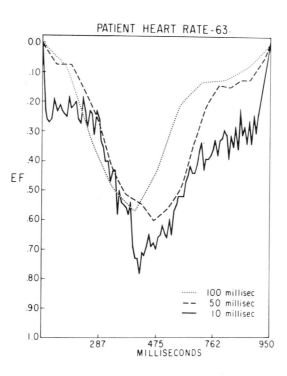

FIG. 1. Ejection fraction curves at three different counting intervals in a patient studied with a heart rate of 63.

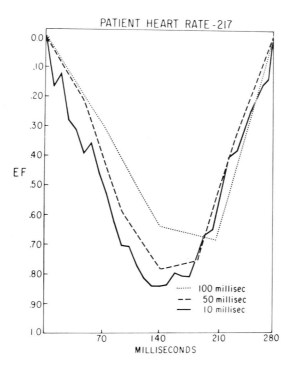

FIG. 2. These left ventricular curves in a patient with a heart rate of 217 were obtained at three different counting intervals.

The relationship of optimal counting intervals (OCI) to heart rate (HR) was determined by linear regression to be OCI = 37 - .11 X HR (Fig. 5). These data indicate the optimal counting interval for obtaining left ventricular volume curves to be less than 50 msec for all heart rates. At rapid heart rates, the inaccuracy of lower counts never exceeds the increased accuracy of high temporal resolution, and the curve never reaches a minimum. At heart rates less than 150, decreasing the counting interval to less than 30 msec does not provide enough improvement in measuring the biologic process to offset the deterioration of data resulting from the lower counts in the data.

The mean percent error in ejection fraction for the low, medium and high heart rate groups is shown in Fig. 6. These data also illustrate the relatively greater importance of using a shorter counting interval as the heart rate increases. The slow heart rate group has the lowest mean error over a wide range of counting intervals and reaches a minimum at the 30 msec interval. The mean error for the medium heart rate group also reaches a minimum at 30 msec. Moreover, the error in ejection fraction at counting intervals shorter or longer than 30 msec increases more markedly in this group than in the low heart rate group. The error in the high heart rate group consistently decreases as the counting interval is shortened from 100 to 10 msec and reaches a minimum at the shortest interval tested.

Visual inspection of images of the left ventricle at different counting intervals identified the most brief counting interval which provided images of sufficient quality to permit volume determinations. Patients studied with a heart rate less than 100 required counting intervals of 40 msec or greater to consistently provide acceptable left ventricular images. The minimum counting interval providing acceptable images in patients studied with a heart rate between 100 and 150 was 30 msec. A 20-msec counting interval was required to provide images of the left ventricle in patients studied with heart rates greater than 150.

DISCUSSION

Radionuclide cardiac studies have been performed using electrocardiographic gating of acquired data and using the initial transit of tracer through the heart. A major advantage of gated studies is that many sequential determinations can be performed. Radionuclide angiocardiograms obtained from the initial transit of tracer provide hemodynamic measurements and permit assessment of left ventricular function. Moreover, the low background in adjacent cardiac chambers inherent with radionuclide angiocardiography provides an outline of the entire ventricle which permits accurate calculation of actual chamber volumes. The counting rate obtained during the first transit of tracer through the heart greatly influences the accuracy of radionuclide angiocardiography. Count-rate limitations become particularly severe in studies performed during exercise with a rapid heart rate and brief transit of tracer through the central circulation. All radionuclide angiocardiograms performed in this study were acquired using the Baird-Atomic System Seventy-Seven which is the most sensitive gamma camera system currently available. This instrument has a maximum counting rate of 380,000 counts per second and studies performed using 15 mCi of technetium-99m pertechnetate in the present investigation achieved an average counting rate of 300,000 counts per second.

VENTRICULAR OUTLINE AND END-SYSTOLIC IMAGE
Patient Heart Rate = 66

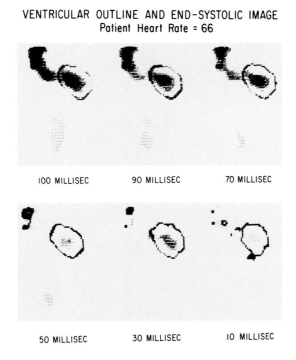

100 MILLISEC   90 MILLISEC   70 MILLISEC

50 MILLISEC   30 MILLISEC   10 MILLISEC

FIG. 3. These end-diastolic parameters about the end-systolic image were obtained from data at different count intervals.

VENTRICULAR OUTLINE AND END-SYSTOLIC IMAGE
Patient Heart Rate = 184

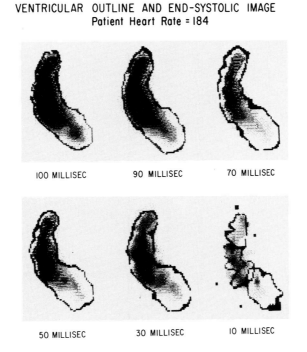

100 MILLISEC   90 MILLISEC   70 MILLISEC

50 MILLISEC   30 MILLISEC   10 MILLISEC

FIG. 4. These images of end-diastolic parameter about the end-systolic counts were obtained at different counting intervals in a patient studied at a heart rate of 184 beats per minute.

Data recorded by the Baird-Atomic System Seventy-Seven gamma camera
is accumulated in a buffer memory and transferred to disc in binary
form. The time necessary for buffer storage and data transfer have
previously limited count accumulation intervals to a minimum of 50 msec.
In two separate experiments, we have documented the accuracy of ejection
fraction and end-diastolic volume measurements obtained with the Baird-
Atomic System Seventy-Seven using the software for evaluation of the
left ventricle (Volume II). In one group of patients, radionuclide
studies were performed immediately prior to cardiac catheterization. In a
second group of subjects, dye indicator dilution cardiac outputs were
compared to radionuclide outputs obtained from volumetric techniques
applied to the left ventricular data. A close correlation in both
studies suggests intrinsic accuracy of the radionuclide technique.

Evaluation of cardiac performance during the stress of exercise
appears to provide clinically useful information in patients with cardiac
disorders. Patients with ischemic heart disease often have normal
cardiac function at rest, but respond to exercise by cardiac dilatation(6,7).
Radionuclide angiocardiograms have been performed during exercise at
heart rates exceeding 220 beats per minute. At these rapid heart rates,
the entire cardiac cycle lasts for less than 300 msec. The period of
end-systole may be quite brief and counting intervals of 50 msec would
not accurately reflect the end-systolic volume. Because of the potential
error in left ventricular volume measurements at rapid heart rates, the
Baird-Atomic System Seventy-Seven gamma camera was modified to operate
at counting intervals as brief as 10 msec. The speed of disc rotation
and quantity of data transferred permits data from four counting intervals
to be recorded during a single disc revolution. Therefore, each 10-msec
period of data acquisition is separated by 2 msec required for data
recording. At counting intervals of 20 msec or greater, only 1 msec is
required for data storage.

The present study was undertaken to determine the optimal counting
interval at different heart rates. Progressively decreasing the duration
of the count accumulation should enhance the accuracy of definition of
the continuously changing left ventricular volume. However, the decrease
in counting interval results in a concomitant decrease in counts accumulated
since the maximum counting rate which may be achieved is determined by
the sensitivity of the gamma camera. Until instrumentation with much
higher maximum counting rates is developed, the accuracy of radionuclide
data reflecting rapid biologic processes will be determined largely by
the total counts achieved. Accurate construction of images reflecting a
distribution of radioactivity requires a greater number of counts than
are required when data from detector areas are grouped for curve generation.
Thus, the optimal counting interval for defining the left ventricular
volume curve is more brief than the optimal counting interval for
imaging left ventricular wall motion.

The results in this report are relevant only to radionuclide angiocardiogram data recorded at a counting rate of 300,000 counts per second.
Studies recorded with a lower maximum counting rate would require longer
counting intervals to achieve equivalent accuracy. Moreover, these data
suggest that accurate radionuclide angiocardiograms would be difficult
to obtain in patients with heart rates greater than 150 using gamma
cameras with a maximum counting rate less than 100,000 counts per second.
Electrocardiogram gating of acquired cardiac images obtained following
equilibrium of a blood pool tracer remains independent of constraints

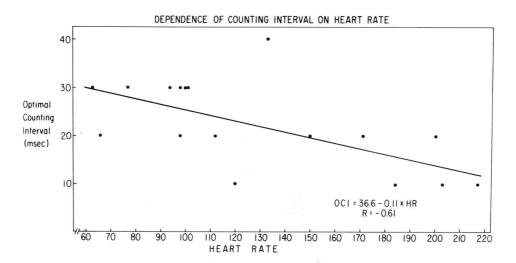

FIG. 5. The optimal counting interval for construction of left ventricular volume curves decreases with increasing heart rate.

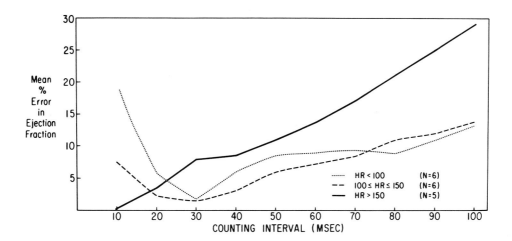

FIG. 6. The mean percent error in ejection fraction determination at each counting interval is compared for three groups of patients separated by heart rate.

imposed by sensitivity of the gamma camera. Data describing the optimal counting interval for radionuclide angiocardiogram definition of left ventricular function are not directly applicable to gated cardiac studies.

Definition of the optimum counting interval in this study was determined as a compromise between two conflicting influences. The interval short enough to reflect closely the left ventricular volume change, but long enough to provide statistically reliable data was considered optimal. In clinical practice, considerations such as the quantity of data which must be stored and the increased operator time necessary to process the larger amounts of data may also be important. Moreover, error introduced by longer counting intervals exerts a consistent influence on ejection fraction measurement. Increasing the counting interval tends to decrease the difference between end-diastolic and end-systolic counts thereby causing an ejection fraction less than the actual value. Because many programs for background subtraction have been somewhat arbitrarily defined by comparison with cardiac catheterization data, the consistent bias resulting from long counting intervals has often been compensated for by excessive background subtraction. The magnitude of error introduced in the ejection fraction measurement for studies in patients with heart rates less than 150 remains below 15% of the actual ejection fraction for all counting intervals. The ejection fraction does not need to be measured with high precision to be clinically relevant. Therefore, left ventricular function may be evaluated appropriately using longer counting intervals than defined to be optimal by this study.

However, radionuclide angiocardiogram evaluation of left ventricular function in patients with heart rates greater than 150 requires counting intervals of 50 msec or less to maintain ejection fraction measurements with less than 10% error. Moreover, comparison of a rest and exercise ejection fraction in a patient studied at two heart rates, but with the same counting interval would tend to underestimate the ejection fraction at the higher heart rate. The increasing use of rest and exercise radionuclide angiocardiogram data emphasizes the importance of selecting the appropriate counting interval for data acquisition. Our experience suggests that evaluation of cardiac function at rest and exercise will provide a large amount of useful clinical information. Instrumentation with brief count accumulation intervals and high sensitivity is necessary for accurate evaluation of left ventricular performance at the high heart rates which occur at maximum exercise.

REFERENCES

1. Kirch, D.L., Metz, C.E., Steele, P.P.: Quantitation of Valvular Insufficiency by Computerized Radionuclide Angiocardiography. Am J Cardiol 34: 711-21, 1974.

2. Jones, R.H., Sabiston, D.C. et al.: Quantitative Radionuclide Angiocardiography for Determination of Chamber to Chamber Transit Times. Am J Cardiol 30: 855-64, 1972.

3. Maltz, D.L., Treves, S.: Quantitative Radionuclide Angiocardiography: Determination of Qp:Qs in Children. Circulation 47: 1049-56, 1973.

4. Anderson, P.A.W., Jones, R.H., and Sabiston, D.C.: Quantitation of Left-to-right Cardiac Shunts with Radionuclide Angiography. Circulation 49: 512-16, 1974.

5. Howe, W.R., Jones, R.H., Sabiston, D.C.: Radionuclide Assessment of LV Function Following Cardiac Surgery. Surgical Forum 27: 1976.

6. Borer, J.S., Bacharach, S.L., Green, M.V. et al.: Real-time Radionuclide Cineangiography in the Non-invasive Evaluation of Global and Regional Left Ventricular Function at Rest and During Exercise in Patients with Coronary Artery Disease. NEJM 296: 296-839, 1977.

7. Rerych, S.K., Scholz, P.M., Newman, G.E., Sabiston, D.C., Jones, R.H.: Cardiac Function at Rest and during Exercise in Normals and in Patients with Coronary Heart Disease: Evaluation by Radionuclide Angiocardiography: Annals of Surgery, In Press.

8. Grenier, R.P., Bender, M.A., Jones, R.H.: A Computerized Multicrystal Scintillation Gamma Camera. In Instrumentation in Nuclear Medicine. Edited by G.J. Hine and J.A. Sorenson. New York, Academic Press, 1974.

9. Jones, R.H., Grenier, R.P., Sabiston, D.C.: Description of a New High Count-rate Gamma Camera System. International Atomic Energy Symposium on Medical Radioisotope Scintigraphy, Monte Carlo, IAEA, Vienna, October 1972.

10. Jones, R.H., Bates, B.B. et al.: Basic Considerations in Computer Use for Dynamic Quantitative Radionuclide Studies. Proceedings of Second Symposium on Sharing of Computer Programs and Techniques in Nuclear Medicine, Oak Ridge, Tennessee, April 21-22, 1972.

11. Jones, R.H., Scholz, P.M.: Data Enhancement Techniques for Radionuclide Cardiac Studies. Medical Radionuclide Imaging 2: 255-66, 1977.

SOURCES OF VIRTUAL BACKGROUND

IN MULTI-IMAGE BLOOD POOL STUDIES

Michael V. Green, Stephen L. Bacharach,
Margaret A. Douglas, Jeffrey S. Borer,
and Gerald S. Johnston

National Institutes of Health
Bethesda, Maryland   20014

ABSTRACT

When multi-image ECG-gated equilibrium studies are analyzed by count-rate methods to obtain measures of left ventricular function, several "virtual" background sources can arise that are additive to the already existing ambient radiation background. Two of these sources, due to left ventricular count rate-volume non-linearity and to phase variations during cardiac cycle, are examined.

INTRODUCTION

An accurate and precise determination of left ventricular (LV) back-ground (BKG) is central to the quantitative accuracy of nuclear medicine procedures designed to measure LV function. Background determination is of critical importance because background comprises one of the two components present in every LV time-activity curve (TAC). One component can be attri-buted to activity that resides in the LV, and the second component (back-ground) can be attributed to activity seen within the LV region-of-interest but actually exterior to the LV. Since, in the TAC, these two components present themselves in summed form, each TAC must be corrected for BKG before LV function can be determined. Moreover, when the magnitude of this BKG represents a large fraction of the total TAC counts, as it does in multi-image equilibrium studies, the accuracy of the BKG determination sets the overall accuracy of the method.

Since BKG traditionally has been viewed as originating entirely outside the LV, it has been assumed that BKG can be found in principle by determin-ing the count rate in some non-LV region in the vicinity of the heart. Moreover, it has also been assumed that this BKG is time-independent and spatially homogeneous or exists with some predefined functional form over the LV region.

While BKG correction schemes based on these assumptions clearly indi-cate that radioactivity external to the ventricle does in fact comprise a large proportion of BKG, more detailed consideration suggests that ambient external activity is not the only possible source. Indeed, several "vir-tual" BKG sources can be identified that arise not from radioactivity ex-ternal to the LV but which can be attributed to violations of the two major assumptions on which multi-image methods are based: (1) that exter-nal LV count rate is absolutely proportional to LV volume and (2) that each cardiac cycle mechanically resembles every other cardiac cycle. Since the magnitude of such "virtual" BKGs cannot, by definition, be determined merely by identifying a BKG region in the patient, an appreciation of the magnitude of such BKGs is necessary if an optimum BKG correction strategy is to be formulated.

COUNT RATE-LV VOLUME LINEARITY

Though over the ranges usually encountered clinically, count rate and volume bear a _relatively_ linear relationship, detailed analysis demonstra-tes that variation from linearity must occur to some extent. The LV blood mass, which in itself constitutes an absorber and scatterer, is embedded in a tissue mass of varying physical properties. This blood and tissue aggregation absorbs and scatters radiation according to the depth of the source within this mass. Since some source points are further from the detector than others, and therefore shielded by larger amounts of tissue, a gradient in detection sensitivity must exist along the line of sight through the ventricle. (external activity around the ventricle is, of course, also modulated by this gradient.)

The potential magnitude of this effect can be roughly calculated by a consideration of cardiac geometry. Figure 1 portrays an anatomic cross-section through the chest at about the mid-ventricular level. As suggested in the figure the ventricle is assumed to be viewed by a detector placed in a 30-40° left anterior oblique projection. If now a point source of ^{99m}Tc is located at the ventricular apex and an attenuation coefficient equal to water is assumed (0.15/cm), only about 50% of the counts emitted by this source will be detected compared to the count rate for this source if it were located at the skin surface. If the source is moved "back" to the mitral valve, only about 25% of the skin surface rate will be observed. Thus, with this model, detection sensitivity varies by a factor of two from the "front" to the back of the ventricle.

As a consequence of this variation in detection sensitivity, when the LAO view is used, activity in the left atrium will be preferentially suppressed as compared with activity in the (nearer) LV. Since the left atrium partially overlaps the LV in the straight LAO projection, this fact may in part explain why studies in the LAO (1) and in the modified LAO projections (2) produce similar quantitative results. However, another consequence of the variation in detection sensitivity is that the relative detection efficiency for large and small LVs may not be the same, either from patient to patient or, more importantly, in the same patient at end diastole (ED) and end systole (ES).

The effect of this non-linearity (which has been deliberately exaggerated for purposes of this discussion) is illustrated in Figure 2 for two "ventricles" (A and B), both possessing the same stroke volume (100 ml) but different ED volumes (175 and 300 ml respectively.) Over each stroke volume range it is clear that count rate is nearly proportional to volume. However, if each of these linear segments is extrapolated back through zero volume, two non-zero intercepts arise, B_1 and B_2. These intercepts are equivalent to an additional BKG component, i.e., a "virtual" BKG. That is, if LV BKG due to all other sources were exactly compensated, an additional increment of BKG in the amounts B_1 and B_2 would have to be made to ventricles A and B in order that the count-determined EFs agree with the volume determined EFs. The effect of count-volume non-linearity on the A and B EFs is shown in the table inset to the figure. This source of virtual BKG is seen to increase with ED volume and with diminishing stroke volume (or EF). The "worst case," therefore, would be expected to arise in patients with grossly dilated and failing ventricles. In the presence of perfect BKG correction from all other sources, however, the effect should give rise to a chronic underestimate in "true" EF over the entire volume range.

When actual measurements (in air) are made in prolate spheroid phantoms (2:1 major/minor axis ratio) or spheres of known volume, a non-linear count-volume is indeed observed. Moreover, if the major axis of the spheroids is tilted away from the detector and all spheroids are measured at this angle, a set of slightly different non-linear relationships is obtained, one for each viewing angle. These results suggest that count-volume non-linearities may exist that depend on viewing angle, absolute ED volume and EF, and in all probability, on ventricular shape.

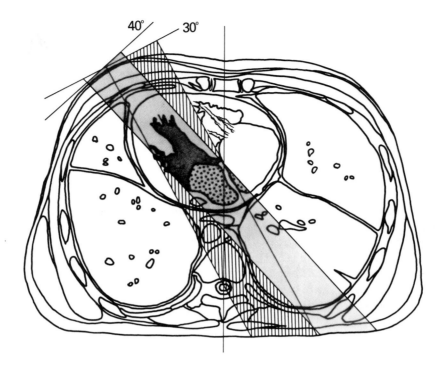

FIG. 1. Cross sectional anatomy at the mid-ventricular level.

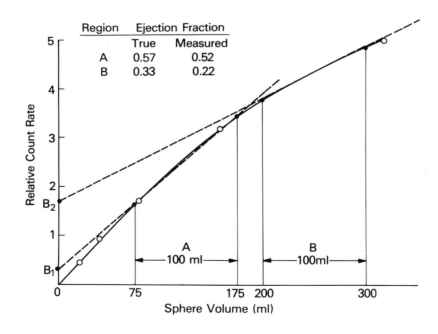

FIG. 2. Effect of count rate-volume non-linearity. B_1 and B_2 are virtual backgrounds.

However, in these same phantom studies, it was also observed that by immersing the phantom in scattering material the linearity between count rate and volume was improved. Moreover, a similar response was noted if the pulse height analyzer "window" was opened to increase acceptance of scattered radiation. In concert, these results suggest that "true" absorption events, which remove photons from the detector's view, can be partially compensated by accepting photons that in the presence of scattering material are now directed into the detector. Since the LV exists in a scattering environment, count-volume linearity may actually be somewhat better in patients than indicated by phantom studies in air.

HEART-RATE (PHASE) FLUCTUATIONS

Among the most difficult problems associated with multi-image studies, both from an experimental and theoretical point of view, is that associated with attempts to discern the effects of fluctuations in the duration of the principle subcycle events: systole, early diastolic filling, diastasis and atrial contraction. If the temporal variations in these intervals from beat-to-beat are appreciable, it follows that superimposition of many such beats will result in a TAC that does not correctly portray LV volume variations. For example, if two LV volume curves are summed, both with the same EF and ED volume, but with different systolic intervals, the resultant curve will exhibit a reduced EF. This reduction in EF is again completely equivalent to the addition of a "virtual" BKG component to the already existing ambient radiation BKG. In this case, virtual BKG arises from an interaction between dynamical behavior of the heart and the (high temporal resolution) reconstruction process used to create the multi-image sequence.

Variations in the lengths of the various sub-intervals are, in fact, known to exist. For example, the relationship between the duration of systole and mean heart rate is used for diagnostic purposes in phono-cardiography. Since patients in the steady state also exhibit <u>fluctuations</u> in heart rate, it is reasonable to assume that some or all of the aforementioned intervals vary in length to some extent with each beat. Unfortunately, the variations in these intervals on a beat-by-beat basis are not well known. As a result, indirect methods have been used to estimate these variations.

One approach to obtaining these estimates is shown in Figure 3. Here the duration of systole (R-wave to minimum in LV TAC) is plotted against mean beat length for two groups of patients studied scintigraphically at rest. The first group consisted of 63 patients with cardiac disease. The data points and information in the figure refer to this group. The regression line to these data is so labelled. The second group studied scintigraphically consisted of 20 normal volunteers free of cardiac (or other) disease. The regression relation obtained in this group is labelled N(20). The third regression relation shown in the figure (N(HWB)23) was obtained by Hammermeister, et al. by measuring the time from maximum to minimum volume as determined from high frame rate contrast angiographic studies performed in 23 normal patients (3).

The slope of the regression equation obtained in the disease group (0.18) suggests that the systolic interval will typically vary by 18 msec/100 msec variation in mean beat length. Since, however, the normal scintigraphic and contrast regression lines do not differ appreciably over the normal beat length range and the contrast values were obtained for single beats, it would appear reasonable to attribute an 18-msec variation in systolic length to a 100-msec variation in (single) beat length. That is, we conceive of the measurements shown in the figure as representing measurements made in a single (composite) "individual" at 63 different instantaneous heart rates. When similar regression lines are obtained for the other intervals, the following variations are found: systole (as noted): 18 msec/100 msec; early diastolic filling: 12 msec/100 msec; diastasis: 58 msec/100 msec and atrial contraction: 4 msec/100 msec.

Thus, if these values do represent the approximate sub-interval variations occurring in a typical individual we could conclude that only the diastasis interval varies sufficiently with beat length to importantly influence high temporal resolution TACs. With the subject at rest the first two-thirds of the cardiac cycle (systole and early diastolic filling) appear to be essentially time stationary and could thus be superimposed without introducing a virtual BKG of any consequence. Provisions must be made, however, to construct the last third of the cycle in such a way as to reflect the large variations in the diastasis interval. (Framing backward in time from the R-wave appears to be one solution to this problem (4).

It is not enough, however, to know just the variation in these sub-interval lengths as a function of beat length. One must also know how beat length fluctuations are distributed in a typical patient population. (If, for example, all patients exhibited a 200-msec variation in beat length then all the ratios above would be multiplied by two and the effect would take on much greater significance.)

To obtain information regarding the distribution of beat length fluctuations throughout a population, beat length distribution functions (number of beats vs. beat length) were constructed in 112 patients studied at rest. A typical distribution for one patient is shown in Figure 4. The full width of this distribution at its half maximum value (FWHM) was taken as a measure of beat length fluctuation for that patient.

Figure 5 represents the relationship between the number of patients per 20-msec FWHM interval and FWHM. This result suggests that beat length fluctuations are distributed over the patient population in a Poisson-like fashion, with some 87% of patients exhibiting variations of less than 110 msec and 13%, more than 110 msec. Thus, in about 87% of patients, sub-interval variations less than or equal to those listed previously would be expected, while in the remaining 13%, greater variations would be expected. In a statistical sense it does not appear that beat length fluctuations introduce a significant virtual BKG in the great majority of patients. The possibility exists, however, that such fluctuations could cause occasional distortion of LV TACs in patients with extremely low heart rates.

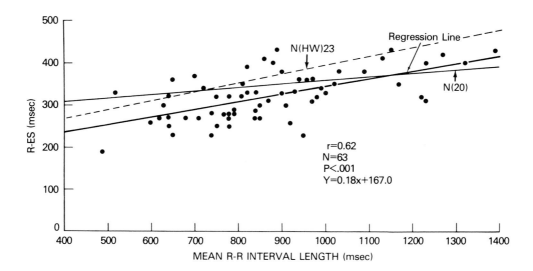

FIG. 3. Scintigraphic relationship between systolic interval length and beat length in 63 patients with disease and in 20 normal volunteers (N(20)); similar measurements by contrast methods (N(HW)23) are shown.

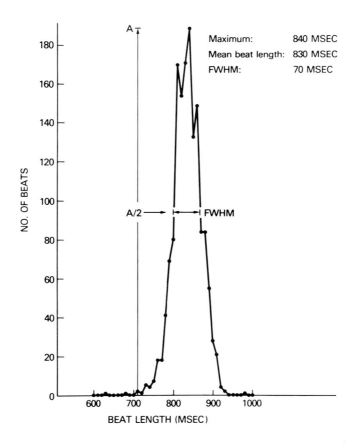

FIG. 4. Beat length distribution function obtained in a typical patient at rest. Beat length fluctuation is measured by FWHM.

If FWHM is plotted against beat length for this same patient group, an estimate of the effect of gross changes in heart rate on these sub-interval variations can be obtained (Fig. 6). The regression equation to these data indicates that a 10-msec <u>decrease</u> in the width of the beat length distribution function occurs for each 100-msec decrease in beat length, i.e., beat length fluctuations become absolutely smaller with increasing heart rate. If all the regression relations obtained in these patients (at rest) are extrapolated for heart rates observed during exercise, these data (Fig. 6) suggest that in the exercise state fluctuations in sub-cycle events should be even less significant (including the diastasis interval which ultimately disappears at high heart rates). For example, suppose a patient has a heart rate of 60 beats/min (mean length = 1000 msec) at rest and the patient increases his rate (by exercise) to 120 beats/min (mean length = 500 msec); according to the regression equation in Figure 6, FWHM will fall from 78 msec at rest to 32 msec during exercise. Based on the foregoing arguments, the total variation in systolic length (for example) would fall from 14 msec at rest to 6 msec during exercise, a negligible variation.

SUMMARY

Total LV BKG can be understood as consisting of two parts: the first (and undoubtedly most important) arises from activity external to the LV but seen within the LV region-of-interest. The second component represents the combined effect of all virtual sources. The present work illustrates how, in two cases, a virtual BKG can arise from violation of the assumptions upon which multi-image methods are based.

Empirically, it has been demonstrated that, irrespective of such effects, EFs obtained by standard count-based radionuclide procedures are valid. Recent work by Burow, et al. (1), Parker, et al. (2) and Folland, et al. (5) has clearly shown that EFs obtained (at rest) by count-rate analysis of multi-image studies are in excellent correlation with those obtained by contrast methods (in which only several cardiac cycles are used). Since such studies are necessarily performed in patients with varying heart rates (and heart-rate fluctuations) and over a wide range of ED volumes and EFs, such agreement would not be expected unless virtual BKG were of secondary importance. (It is possible, however, that systematic deviations observed in these studies are, in part, a result of virtual BKG.) Moreover, in rest-exercise studies in which all these variables are altered in the same patient (6) count analysis and geometric analysis of multi-image sequences (in separate studies) has shown similar directional and magnitude changes in EF for the same classes of patients (coronary artery disease and normals). Since geometric analysis does not possess a virtual BKG dependence, this agreement also suggests a secondary role for virtual BKG in count-based studies. In addition, rest-exercise studies performed using first-pass methods have also yielded directional and magnitude changes similar to those observed with equilibrium methods (7). Since only several contiguous cardiac cycles are used in first-pass procedures (rather than hundreds), phase variations do not appear to be of critical importance. A similar interpretation can also be applied to comparative first-pass and equilibrium studies in animals (8) where EFs

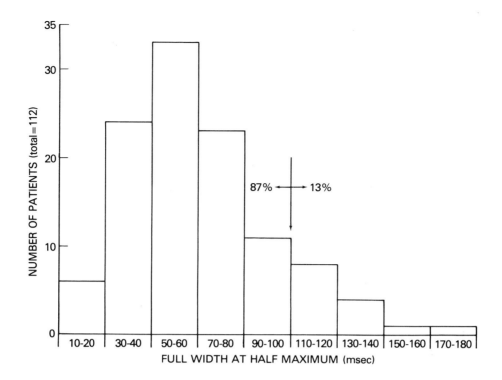

FIG. 5. Distribution of beat length fluctuations for a group of 112 patients at rest.

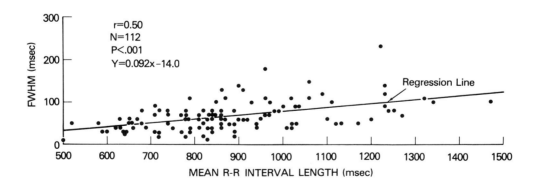

FIG. 6. Relationship between beat length fluctuations and mean beat length. Regression line suggests that such fluctuations diminish with increasing heart rate.

obtained by each method were found to agree over a wide range of heart
rates and cardiac outputs.

The remarkable internal consistency of these (and other) investigations clearly demonstrates the clinical applicability of count-rate analysis of multi-image studies, and by this standard the issue of virtual BKG
is perhaps moot. Nonetheless, such global comparisons cannot, in the end,
provide a wholly satisfying explanation of the detailed effects that might
occur in the presence of virtual BKG. If this issue is to be laid to rest
or, instead, to serve as a guide in formulating a BKG correction strategy
of greater absolute accuracy, much investigational work remains to be done.

ACKNOWLEDGEMENTS

The authors are indebted to Dr Karl E. Hammermeister and his col-
leagues at the Seattle Veterans Administration Hospital for permitting
our use of their original data to obtain the regression line shown in
Figure 3. The authors also wish to express their gratitude to Ms. Bonnie
Mack and to Ms. Susan Farkas for their superb technical support in this
work and to Ms. Luella Bentz for preparing the manuscript.

REFERENCES

1. Burrow RD, Strauss HW, Singleton R, et al: Analysis of left
ventricular function from multiple gated acquisition cardiac blood pool
imaging. Circ 56: 1024-1028, 1977

2. Parker JA, Uren RF, Jones AG, et al: Radionuclide left ventriculography with the slant hole collimator. J Nucl Med 18: 848-851, 1977

3. Hammermeister KE, Brooks RC, Warbasse JR: The rate of change of
left ventricular volume in man. Circ 49: 729-737, 1974

4. Bacharach SL, Green MV, Borer JS, et al: A real-time system for
multi-image gated cardiac studies. J Nucl Med 18: 79-84, 1977

5. Folland ED, Hamilton GW, Larson SM, et al: The radionuclide
ejection fraction: a comparison of three radionuclide techniques with
contrast angiography. J Nucl Med 18: 1159-1166, 1977

6. Borer JS, Bacharach SL, Green MV, et al: Real time radionuclide
cineangiography in the noninvasive evaluation of global and regional left
ventricular function at rest and during exercise in patients with coronary
artery disease. New Eng J Med 296: 839-844, 1977

7. Jengo JA, Uzler M, Conant R, et al: Exercise stress first-pass
radionuclide LV function (ejection fraction and segmental wall motion).
This proceedings.

8. Fletcher JW, Herbig FK, Daly JL, et al: Measurement and comparison of left ventricular ejection fraction utilizing first transit gated
scintigraphy. Proceedings: Fifth Symposium on Sharing Computer Programs
and Technology in Nuclear Medicine, Salt Lake City, Utah. CONF-750124,
1975. Technical Information Service, Springfield, Va.

THE EFFECT OF ERRORS IN DETERMINING LEFT VENTRICULAR EJECTION FRACTION FROM RADIONUCLIDE COUNTING DATA

David L. Williams, Ph.D.; and Glen W. Hamilton, M. D.

Veterans Administration Hospital
Nuclear Medicine Section
Seattle, Washington 98108

ABSTRACT

The influence on calculated ejection fraction of statistical and systematic errors in the measured count values at end-diastole and end-systole has been studied. It is found that the relative contribution of the various errors depends strongly on the patient's true ejection fraction and on the radionuclide measurement technique used to determine it. Neither the first-transit nor equilibrium blood-pool methods are clearly superior from an error-analysis viewpoint.

INTRODUCTION

Quantitative methods for determining left ventricular end-diastolic volume (EDV) and end-systolic volume (ESV) by cineradiography and radionuclide studies are frequently used to measure left ventricular performance. The fractional volume of blood ejected per beat or systolic ejection fraction (EF) is commonly used as a measure of overall ventricular function.

Ejection fraction is defined as the ratio of stroke volume (SV) to end-diastolic volume:

$$EF = \frac{SV}{EDV} = \frac{EDV - ESV}{EDV}$$

Based on this mathematical relationship, it is possible to estimate the deviation of ejection fraction from its true value when errors are made in the primary determination of EDV, ESV, or both, by using the theory of error propagation. Calculation and graphic display of the influence of these errors upon the EF has proved useful in developing strategies to minimize error and to improve the reliability of radiographic and radionuclide studies.

It is conventional to characterize the sources of error as either statistical or systematic. As expected, the statistical uncertainty in EF is reduced as the number of acquired counts increases. In contrast, systematic errors such as those produced by incorrect definition of areas-of-interest or incorrect specification of background are more serious, since they cannot be reduced simply by acquiring more data. The next sections summarize the influence these sources of error have on the calculated ejection fraction obtained from nuclear counting data.

METHODS

In Appendix I, the theory of error propagation is used to establish a relationship between errors in end-diastolic counts (EDC) and end-systolic counts (ESC) to errors in EF under the assumption that the uncertainties in EDC and ESC are independent (I-5). To examine the effects that statistical variations in EDC and ESC have upon uncertainty in EF, the error propagation equation was evaluated under the condition that Poisson statistics govern the variability in these measured quantities. Equation I-10 in the appendix expresses the fractional statistical uncertainty in the ejection fraction as a function of EF and EDC:

$$\frac{\sigma EF}{EF} = \frac{1}{EF} \sqrt{\frac{(1-EF)\ (2-EF)}{EDC}}$$

The value of EDC required to measure a known ejection fraction, EF, to a specified statistical accuracy, ($\sigma EF/EF$), is obtained by a simple rearrangement of terms (Eq. I-11):

$$EDC = \frac{(1-EF)\ (2-EF)}{EF^2\ \left(\frac{\sigma EF}{EF}\right)^2}$$

     To study the effects of systematic errors in EDC and ESC, arbitrary
values of these parameters were chosen to result in true EF's of 0.15, 0.33,
0.50, 0.67, and 0.80. Errors ranging from ± 5% to ± 80% were then introduced
into the EDC, ESC, or both, and the resultant EF calculated.

RESULTS

Statistical Errors

     The effect of statistical variability in the measured values of EDC and
ESC is obtained by numerical evaluation of Equation I-11 and is illustrated
in Fig. 1. It is observed that statistical variations are much more severe
at low ejection fractions, requiring approximately ten times as many counts
at a low EF (0.2) than at a high EF (0.6) to achieve the same statistical
accuracy. The difficulty in measuring a low EF is essentially a problem of
accurately estimating the difference between two noisy quantities (EDC and
ESC) whose mean values differ by a small amount.

     The difficulty in making first-transit measurements of EF with the
Anger camera, due to statistical errors, is readily apparent. Peak left
ventricular counts range between 10^2 and 10^4, with statistical errors between
10% and 40% per cardiac cycle. Gating the first transit study in order to
decrease the uncertainty in EDC and ESC can improve the statistical accuracy
by a factor of 2 or 3 for the composite beat (1). The equilibrium blood-pool
gating techniques provide better control of statistical variability by continually acquiring data until a specified accuracy is achieved. A typical
blood-pool study can acquire 50 K to 100 K counts at end-diastole over a
period of 3-4 minutes, and thus achieve statistical uncertainties of less
than 10% over the entire clinical EF range (see Fig. 1).

Systematic Errors

     The result of systematic error in the measurement of EDC is graphically
illustrated in Fig. 2. As EDC is overestimated, EF increases. Underestimation of EDC decreases the EF. The effect of error in EDC alone is most pronounced at low EF. Errors of up to ± 20% cause relatively minor error in
calculated EF when true EF exceeds 0.6. With a true EF of 0.5, 10-20%
errors cause substantial change in calculated EF and could easily effect the
clinical interpretation. When the true EF is below 0.2, even minor errors
in EDC produce major changes in EF. The latter may not be significant in a
single clinical study, as an EF of 0.1 and 0.2 both denote extremely poor
ventricular function. However, serial studies which show changes from 0.1 to
0.2 should be viewed with skepticism, as minor error in EDC alone could
easily account for this degree of change.

     The errors in EF which result from over- or underestimation of ESC are
shown in Fig. 3. The linear relationship contrasts to errors in EDC alone
(Fig. 2), and demonstrates that ESC over- or underestimation produces changes
in EF by the same absolute amount. As with errors in EDC alone, errors in
ESC cause more significant errors in calculated EF when the true EF is low.

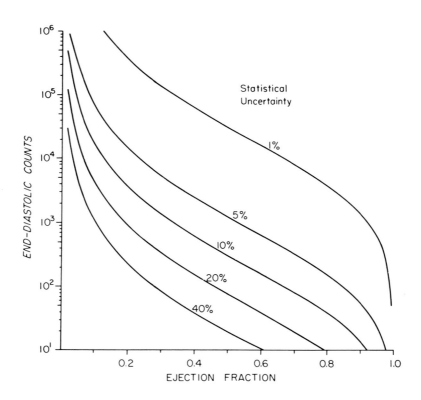

FIG. 1. The influence of statistical errors on the calculated ejection fraction. The end-diastolic counts required to determine a true ejection fraction to a specified statistical uncertainty, as a percentage of the true ejection fraction, are shown.

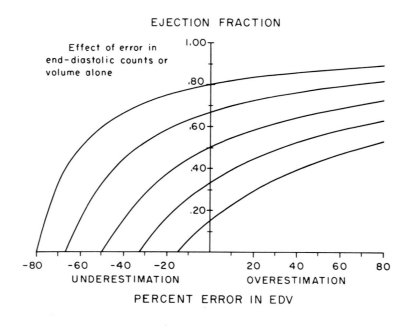

FIG. 2. The effect of systematic error in end-diastolic counts alone.

This type of error is likely the most common error in x-ray-contrast-angiography (see discussion below) and it can cause critical aberrations in calculated EF. When true EF is 0.5, 20% errors in ESC will change the EF from 0.4 to 0.6. The former is clearly abnormal, the latter normal. Due to the pronounced effect of errors at low true ejection fractions, serial studies at low ejection fractions should be interpreted with caution.

Fig. 4 illustrates the situation in which a systematic error of the same absolute amount is present in both EDC and ESC. Overestimation causes a reduction in EF while underestimation produces an increase. In contrast to the two previous cases, the result of systematic error in both EDC and ESC is maximal at high EF and minimal when the EF is low. All radionuclide methods of determining the EF induce this type of error by including non-left ventricular activity in the left ventricular signal; a problem commonly referred to as "background".

Figs. 5 and 6 summarize the combined influence of the three classes of systematic error for the clinical conditions of normal (true EF = 0.66), and severely depressed (true EF = 0.15) ejection fraction. These figures are composed of results taken directly from Figs. 2, 3, and 4. Within the range of $\pm$ 20%, the effect of error in EDC alone and ESC alone are approximately of equal magnitude, and opposite influence. An equal error in both EDC and ESC produces greater error than either error in EDC or ESC alone, when the EF is normal or high. When the EF is low, this type of error effects the EF only slightly.

DISCUSSION

The influence on calculated EF of statistical and systematic errors in the primary measured quantities, EDC, and ESC, has been studied over an EF range of clinical interest. It is apparent from Figs. 1 through 4 that the different types of errors have quite different effects on the EF, and that the magnitude of the resultant error is related to the level of the true EF being measured.

Of the various errors discussed, statistical errors are the most strongly related to the true EF value. A typical first-transit study of the left ventricle contains only about 200-1000 counts at end-diastole; with 1000 EDC's, the statistical uncertainty is 5% at a normal EF and 40% at an EF of 0.10. Mathematical averaging or ECG gating of several cardiac cycles reduces the statistical error slightly but falls far short of the 40,000 counts needed to calculate an EF of 0.10 with 5% uncertainty (see Fig. 1). The much higher count rate afforded by multicrystal imaging devices should make this instrument considerably more accurate for determining low EF's than single crystal devices if all other errors remain equal.

The considerable ventricular dilatation and slow cardiac transit time that usually accompany a low EF also minimize, to a degree, the statistical uncertainty in a low EF. However, even given an EDC count rate of four times normal and twice as many cycles to summate, statistical uncertainty remains rather high when EF is low.

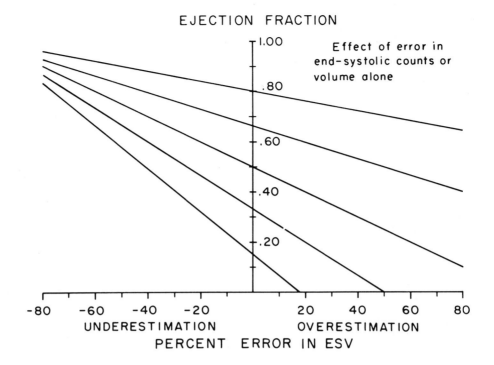

FIG. 3. The effect of systematic error in end-systolic counts alone.

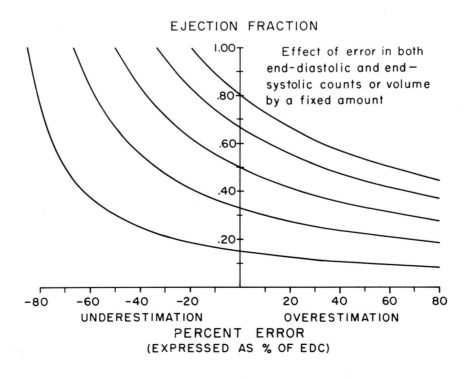

FIG. 4. The effect of systematic errors in end-diastolic and end-systolic counts of the same amount.

Errors in ejection fraction due to over- or underestimation of EDC alone are primarily due to inaccurate definition of the left ventricular region-of-interest. The relatively greater reduction in EF noted with underestimation than the increases noted with overestimation, correlates with the empiric observation of several investigators that a "generous" left ventricular region is preferable to a "skimpy" region as long as contiguous chambers are not included. The relatively stronger effect of EDC errors at low EF's is counteracted by the relative ease with which the low EF, i.e., large volume ventricle, is identified.

Errors in determining ESC (or volume) are a major problem in both radio-nuclide and contrast angiography. In both types of studies, correct identification of left ventricular systolic boundaries is most difficult when the end-systolic volume is small (and EF is normal or high). Fortunately, the effect of errors in ESC is maximal at low, rather than normal or high EF's. In spite of the latter, we believe this error is the major reason why radionuclide techniques employing a fixed region-of-interest for both diastole and systole consistently underestimate normal and high EF's compared to contrast angiography. While this initially seems paradoxical, the magnitude or percent of EDC overestimation due to a fixed region-of-interest is very small when EF is low, because the area change between diastole and systole is small. Conversely, when EF is high, the area change is great and ESC are overestimated by a fixed region-of-interest corresponding to end-diastole. Use of a region-of-interest, which becomes smaller during systole, reduces this type of error if the area change is accurately tracked.

Errors in both EDC and ESC of the same absolute amount are a major problem in radionuclide studies. Almost always this is due to inclusion of counts eminating from adjacent cardiac and non-cardiac structures, i.e., "background". The large magnitude of "background corrections" used to make the EF correspond to contrast angiography makes this a primary source of error in radionuclide studies. It should be stressed that in a typical equilibrium study, the "background level" is often 50% or greater than the left ventricular count rate. Under these circumstances, an EF of 0.33, determined from the uncorrected time-activity curve, becomes 0.67 after background subtraction.

Examination of the likely source of errors at different levels of EF is useful. When EF is normal or high, the most likely error is due to an equal error in both EDC and ESC, i.e., background or the background correction used. The next most likely is error in ESC alone, if a fixed region-of-interest is used. Statistical error and error due to EDC estimation should be minimal. When the EF is low, statistical error is the most likely source of errors in the EF. Both errors in EDC alone and ESC alone have strong effects at low EF levels, but for the reasons discussed, they have much less influence than statistics. Errors due to background will be minimal.

Finally, the errors should be considered in view of the particular radionuclide technique selected. The first-transit technique, by its nature, provides relatively good estimates of EDC and ESC, with minimal background

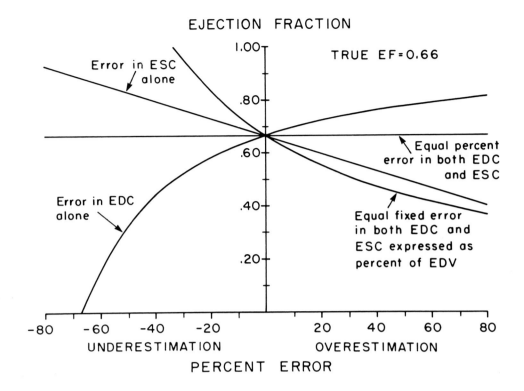

FIG. 5. The combined influence of systematic errors upon a normal (EF = 0.67) ejection fraction.

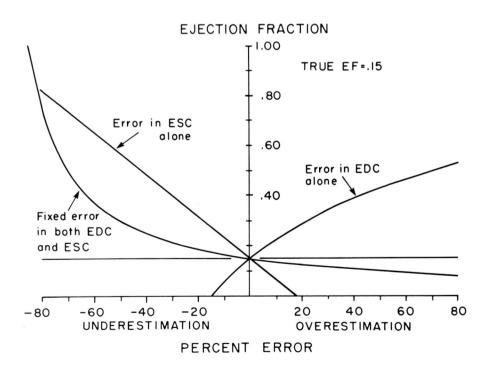

FIG. 6. The combined influence of systematic errors upon a severely depressed (EF = 0.15) ejection fraction.

and usually poor statistics. The equilibrium technique provides good statistics but is much more prone to systematic errors due to inaccurate estimations of EDC, ESC, or both.

CONCLUSION

The influence of statistical and systematic errors in determining end-diastolic and end-systolic counts have been investigated for the ejection fraction range of clinical importance. The magnitude and direction of change in computed EF is highly dependent upon the true EF value and the particular class of error considered. First-transit clinical methods are primarily limited by counting statistics while equilibrium blood-pool techniques are dominated by systematic effects from overlapping and adjacent chambers and vessels. Neither technique is clearly superior from an error-analysis viewpoint.

ACKNOWLEDGEMENTS

This study was supported in part by the Veterans Administration and NHLI Grant #1R01-HL-18805-01. We acknowledge the typing assistance of Mrs. Katharine Jelsing; and the technical assistance of our medical illustrator, Ms. Joy Godfrey, and photographer, Mr. Clinton Kolyer.

REFERENCES

1. Weaver WD, Hamilton GW, Williams DL, et al: Reproducibility of the ejection fraction measured by first-transit radionuclide studies. J Nucl Med 17: 556, 1976 (abst).

2. Evans RD: The Atomic Nucleus. McGraw-Hill, N.Y., 1955, pp. 746-766.

3. Evans RD: The Atomic Nucleus. McGraw-Hill, N.Y., 1955, pp. 766-771.

4. Bevington PR: Data Reduction and Error Analysis for the Physical Sciences. McGraw-Hill, N.Y., 1969, pp. 56-65.

APPENDIX I. Derivation of the Statistical Uncertainty in the Ejection
             Fraction from Counting Data at End-Diastole and End-Systole

In this section, the standard deviation in the ejection fraction for a
single heart cycle (σEF) is derived by considering the statistical error
propagation in the expression:

$$EF = \frac{EDC-ESC}{EDC} \qquad (I-1)$$

where EDC = end-diastolic counts
and ESC = end-systolic counts.

The fractional error in the measured result (σEF/EF) is calculated and
expressed in terms of EDC and EF. Finally, an equation is derived which
specifies the average counts at end-diastole required to measure EF for a
single heart cycle to a specified statistical accuracy.

Consider equation (I-1) where the counts obtained during appropriate
sampling intervals are EDC and ESC at end-diastole and end-systole, respectively. Each are obtained from Poisson distributions which govern radioactive
decay (2). That is, for each sampling interval, the probability $P(n,\mu)$ for
obtaining n counts in one observation when μ is the average over many observations follows from:

$$P(n,\mu) = \frac{\mu^n e^{-\mu}}{n!} \quad [n = 0, 1, 2, \ldots\ldots] \qquad (I-2)$$

The standard deviation in the average counts can be calculated from equation
(I-2), and is well known to be $\sqrt{\mu}$ (2). For a single heart cycle or a composite gated cycle, only one observation can be made at end-diastole and
end-systole, respectively, so that the mean values are estimated to be:

$$\mu(EDC) = EDC \text{ and } \mu(ESC) = ESC$$

The standard deviations in μ(EDC) and μ(ESC) are then given by:

$$\sigma EDC = \sqrt{EDC} \qquad (I-3)$$

$$\sigma ESC = \sqrt{ESC} \qquad (I-4)$$

The error propagation is obtained from an evaluation of the expression
(3,4):

$$\sigma EF^2 = \left(\frac{\delta EF}{\delta EDC}\right)^2 \sigma EDC^2 + \left(\frac{\delta EF}{\delta ESC}\right)^2 \sigma ESC^2 \qquad (I-5)$$

where σEF is the standard deviation in the calculated EF.

It has been assumed that statistical fluctuations in EDC and ESC are uncorrelated. The partial derivatives express the relative importance of

statistical fluctuations in the corresponding variables while the σ's are estimates of the magnitudes of these fluctuations, i.e., the standard deviations. The partial derivatives are calculated to be:

$$\frac{\delta EF}{\delta EDC} = \frac{ESC}{EDC^2} \qquad (I-6)$$

$$\frac{\delta EF}{\delta ESC} = \frac{-1}{EDC} \qquad (I-7)$$

After substitution of equations (I-3), (I-4), (I-6), and (I-7) into equation (I-5), the standard deviation in the ejection fraction is:

$$\sigma EF = \frac{1}{EDC}\sqrt{\frac{ESC}{EDC} \ (EDC + ESC)} \qquad (I-8)$$

- and the relative error in the determination of EF is:

$$\frac{\sigma EF}{EF} = \left(\frac{1}{EDC-ESC}\right)\sqrt{\frac{ESC}{EDC} \ (EDC + ESC)} \qquad (I-9)$$

Equation (I-9) can now be simplified by solving (I-1) for ESC and substituting to obtain:

$$\frac{\sigma EF}{EF} = \frac{1}{EF}\sqrt{\frac{(1-EF) \ (2-EF)}{EDC}} \qquad (I-10)$$

This expression relates the relative statistical error to the true ejection fraction and the count value at end-diastole.

If equation (I-10) is rearranged by solving for EDC, we obtain an expression for the average end-diastolic counts needed to measure a true ejection fraction (EF) to a relative statistical accuracy of $\sigma EF/EF$.

$$\cdot \ EDC = \frac{(1-EF) \ (2-EF)}{EF^2 \ \left(\frac{\sigma EF}{EF}\right)^2} \qquad (I-11)$$

A SYSTEM FOR COMPUTER GENERATION OF LEFT VENTRICULAR MASKS FOR USE IN COMPUTERIZED ECG-GATED RADIONUCLIDE ANGIOCARDIOGRAPHY

Margaret A. Douglas and Michael V. Green

The National Institutes of Health
Bethesda, Md. 20014

ABSTRACT

A procedure for automatic generation of left ventricular (LV) masks for use in computerized radionuclide angiocardiography was designed which sequentially applies six different techniques. Non-moving structures are removed when the ES frame (image) is subtracted from the ED frame. The technique of row and column signatures is applied to the resultant frame (ED-ES) to produce a boxed LV area in the ED. From this frame a computed variable background is subtracted. Next edges are enhanced by locally adapted thresholding. Subsequently this image is pruned by rotating it about its center through three 30-degree rotations; for each rotation those row or column signatures which fall below a fixed threshold are clipped. Finally the rotational artefacts are removed. This procedure has been applied to 20 cases with good results.

INTRODUCTION

Computerized ECG-gated radionuclide angiocardiography has become
increasingly useful in the clinical study of left ventricular function.
Computation of the ejection fraction, however, requires the delineation
of the left ventricle. Generally, an experienced person (e.g. a
cardiologist) delineates the left ventricle by manually outlining and
filling in the left ventricular region of interest (ROI) with a light
pen on a displayed image from the stack of gated cardiac blood pool
frames. This technique has been time consuming and has been a source of
inter-observer variation. The same observer often cannot duplicate his
own outline of a left ventricle on a given cardiac study.

The purpose of this paper is to describe a multiple step
computerized procedure for generating a left ventricle ROI or "mask",
subject to an experienced observer's approval or rejection, which
compares well with the mask as it is currently being manually drawn, and
to discuss our early experiences in applying the mask.

MATERIALS AND METHOD

Radionuclide studies from ten patients were used to develop the
procedure. Six patients had normal LV wall movement and four had
abnormal wall movement. Each study consisted of 30-100 frames (images)
encompassing the entire averaged cardiac cycle obtained by a previously
described method (1). Each frame contained 64 x 64 pixels, with a .5-
centimeter distance from pixel to pixel, and contained the scintillation
image of the heart, great vessels, and surrounding tissues.

The first step is to suppress or remove the scintillation image of
those structures which exhibit no movement. This is achieved by
subtracting the end-systolic image (ES) from the end-diastolic image
(ED). The first five ten-msec frames were summed to compose the ED
image (Fig.1A). Those five consecutive frames which yielded the minimum
sum were summed to compose the ES image (Fig.1B). A nine point
smoothing was applied to the ED and ES images. A positive difference
image was formed by subtraction of the smoothed ES image from the
smoothed ED image and retention of those picture elements greater than
zero (Fig.1C).

The row and column sums of the difference image (ED-ES) are
computed. These signatures are used to establish the borders of the
rectangle encompassing the right and left ventricles. The left border
is determined to be the first column encountered whose sum exceeds 25%
of the peak column sum. The other three borders are determined in a
similar manner.

These four borders are then applied to the ED image (Fig.2A). The
boxed portion of the ED image within the borders is signatured. The
derivative of the smoothed column signatures is used to determine the
discriminating point between the left and right ventricle. If no
discriminator is found, the unsmoothed column signatures are subjected
to successively lighter smoothing and the derivative re-computed. If
these successively lighter smoothings do not result in the locating of a
discriminator, the boxed ED is rotated 45 degrees about its center and

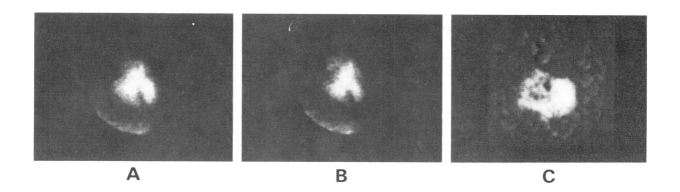

FIG. 1. (A) End-diastolic image; (B) end-systolic image; (C) positive difference image.

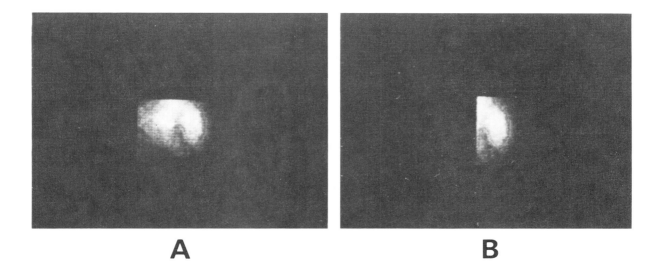

FIG. 2. (A) Boxed ED image; (B) boxed LV image (BLV).

the procedure repeated. At each attempt to locate the discriminator, a
message to that effect is printed on the terminal. If a discriminator
is not located after the rotations, the process is terminated with a
rejection notice.

When the left to right discriminator has been located, the left
ventricle side of the rectangle of the boxed ED image is retained by the
system. This is resignatured to establish a minimum rectangle which
includes all of the left ventricle (Fig.2B). The borders of this boxed
end-diastolic LV (BLV) are used in a technique developed by M. Goris et
al (2) to estimate a variable background mesh (VB).

Creation of this background mesh is accomplished by linear
interpolation of values from border to border along all 45 degree
diagonals from top to left and from top to right borders. The mesh
(Fig.3A) is then subtracted from the boxed ED left ventricle (BLV) image
and the remaining positive picture elements retained as the positive
picture frame (PPF)
(Fig.3B).

$$PPF=BLV-VB.$$

Next a method employing compass gradient masks (3) is used to
enhance left ventricle edges in the positive picture frame. A set of
four orthogonal gradient masks, each enhancing an edge of a given
direction, are convolved with the positive picture frame.

$$C_p(I+1,J+1)= \sum_{K=I}^{I+2} \sum_{L=J}^{J+2} PPF(K,L)*MASK_p(K+1-I,L+1-J) ,$$
$$p=1,\ldots,4.$$

A gradient matrix is formed by using, at each picture element location,
the maximum of the four values produced by the set of orthogonal masks.

$$GRAD(I,J)=MAX \left| C_p(I,J) \right|, p=1,\ldots,4 .$$

This is divided on a point by point basis by the matrix formed by a nine
point smoothing of the positive picture frame (SM) to produce a locally
adaptive threshold matrix (LAT) (Fig.3C).

$$SM(I,J)=1/16 \left[4*PPF(I,J)+PPF(I-1,J-1)+PPF(I-1,J+1) \right.$$
$$+PPF(I+1,J+1)+2*(PPF(I-1,J)+PPF(I,J\_1)+PPF(I,J+1)$$
$$\left. +PPF(I+1,J)) \right]$$

$$LAT(I,J)=GRAD(I,J)/SM(I,J).$$

This LAT matrix is subtracted from the smoothed positive picture frame
(SM) and positive picture elements are retained to produce the edge
corrected frame (ECF) (Fig.3D).

$$ECF(I,J)=SM(I,J)-LAT(I,J).$$

Spurious and isolated pixels are then removed from the ECF in the following manner. The edge corrected frame is rotated 45 degrees about its center. Those rows or columns whose signatures fall below a fixed threshold, expressed as a percentage of the peak row or column signature, are clipped off. Next the picture is rotated about its center through three 30-degree rotations. At the end of each rotation, only those rows and columns whose signatures are greater than a fixed threshold are summed into a master picture file (MPF) in their original orientation. After three 30-degree rotations, a residual background computed as 20% of the average count in non zero pixels of the MPF is subtracted from each element in the MPF to remove artefacts generated by the rotational procedures described above. All remaining positive values are set to one and all non-positive values are set to zero. This becomes the left ventricle mask (Fig. 4).

RESULTS

A set of 20 test cases was used to verify the computer generated LV masks. Verification was accomplished in two ways. The first method was to locate and count the number of pixels by which the automated mask differed from its manually drawn counterpart. Results of this comparison are shown in Table 1. Three cases out of the twenty gave unacceptably large total errors when expressed as a percentage of the number of cells in the drawn mask. In case number 1 the system issued a warning that difficulty was encountered in locating the left to right discriminator. Inspection by an observer indicated that this was caused by a very large right ventricle which resulted in poor left to right separation and the automated mask was rejected. In case number 5 the shape of the automated mask is unusual in that it includes, in addition to LV area, a large bulb shaped projection in the left apical region. This distortion was immediately obvious to an observer and was therefore rejected. In case number 14 the automated mask was significantly larger than its drawn counterpart, particularly at the top of the LV. This difference would not necessarily be detected by an observer and therefore, for the purposes of evaluating the results of the automated system, this mask was not rejected. The average discrepancy for the twenty cases, expressed as a percent of the number of cells in the drawn LV mask was 26.5%. This discrepancy was the result of an 18.2% average over-estimation and an 8.3% under-estimation of the LV mask by the automated system. A second trained observer was employed to draw a second set of LV masks for the same 20 cases. The average discrepancy of these masks versus those of the first observer was 16.8%, consisting of a 13.1% average over-estimation and a 3.1% under-estimation. The average discrepancy between the automated masks and those of the second observer was 26.6%, consisting of a 13.6% over-estimation and a 13.0% under- estimation by the automated system.

A second method of verification used was to generate raw and background corrected time functions using both the automated and the manually drawn LV masks. From these time functions ejection fractions (EF) were computed via

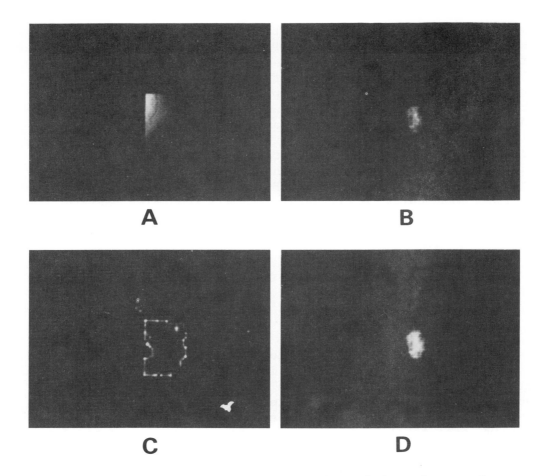

FIG. 3. (A) Variable background mesh (VB); (B) positive picture frame: PPF = BLV - VB; (C) locally adapted threshold (LAT); (D) edge corrected frame: ECF = PPF - LAT.

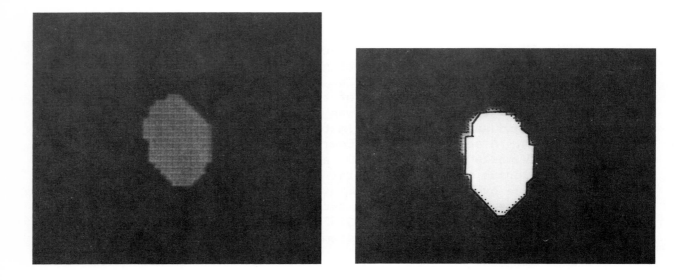

FIG. 4. (Left) Computer generated LV mask; (Right) automated LV mask (....) vs. manually drawn LV mask (----).

$$EF = \frac{ED \text{ volume} - ES \text{ volume}}{ED \text{ volume} - B}$$

where B=average background * number of cells in LV mask.

The background regions for the manually drawn masks were drawn as a crescent in the left apical region, approximately one cell out from the LV mask and one cell in width. The background regions for the automated masks were computer generated as a crescent in the left apical region one cell out from the LV mask. The crescent extended from a point one cell below the midpoint of the base of the LV mask to a point one cell to the right of the LV mask and one third of the distance from the top of the LV mask. The width used for the crescent was either one or two cells, the width being determined as that one which yielded the highest average background value. The results of the automated versus the drawn procedures of EF computation are shown in Table 2. As expected those three cases which showed the highest levels of discrepancy in the previous table comparing mask pixels also showed high levels of difference in EF. The correlation for computed versus drawn mask's EF for the 20 cases was .88. Excluding the two cases in which the automated mask was rejected by the operator, the correlation coefficent for the remaining 18 cases was .98 (Fig.5). EF computed using LV masks and background crescents drawn by a second observer were also compared to those computed using the LV masks and background crescents drawn by the first observer. This yielded a correlation of .97 (Fig.6). Ejection fractions computed by the first observer two to three years ago were compared to his recently computed ejection fractions. These yielded a correlation of .96 (Fig.7).

Finally the background corrected time functions generated by the automated technique and by the manually drawn technique were compared. A point by point comparison of the computed versus drawn mask's time function gave a correlation of at least .99 in each of the cases. A comparison of the peak ejection rate normalized by the end-diastolic volume of the computed versus drawn mask's time functions gave a correlation of .96 for the 18 masks accepted by the operator (Fig.8).

DISCUSSION

The automated generation of LV masks is not infallible. The system must include an observer to either accept or reject the generated mask before its subsequent use. Also, thresholds used in the clipping procedures are probably dependent on the count levels in the summed ED and ES images used. In our case these images typically exhibited more than 300K counts. Our early experience in applying this procedure indicates that, given the above considerations, it generates masks which compare well to those manually drawn. It is rapid, taking an average of 21 seconds of CPU time per mask generated, and should give good reproducibility. Masks generated by this system have a rate of acceptance by the observer of greater than 30%. Differences between the automated mask and its drawn counterpart are comparable both to the differences between masks drawn by two observers and to masks drawn by a

Table 2.   EJECTION FRACTION

| Case No. | Manually Drawn Masks | | | Automated Masks |
	Obs.1 1977	Obs.2 1977	Obs.1 1975	
1	.83	.80	.69	.58
2	.16	.13	.20	.14
3	.51	.50	.55	.48
4	.51	.54	.66	.53
5	.77	.66	.72	.44
6	.46	.50	.51	.43
7	.45	.49	.47	.45
8	.67	.76	.68	.68
9	.63	.72	.65	.63
10	.53	.55	.59	.53
11	.54	.56	.58	.53
12	.66	.77	.68	.70
13	.61	.63	.68	.59
14	.76	.73	.71	.64
15	.46	.48	.48	.43
16	.15	.15	.19	.15
17	.91	1.0	.86	.89
18	.38	.41	.43	.39
19	.43	.46	.42	.43
20	.48	.51	.53	.47
Mean	.55	.57	.56	.51
S.Dev.	.19	.20	.16	.17

Table 1.   COMPARISON OF FIRST OBSERVER'S MASKS VERSUS THOSE OF OBSERVER 2 AND THOSE OF AUTOMATED SYSTEM

| Case No. | No. Cells in Mask Drawn | | | No. Cells Difference vs. Observer 1 | | % Difference vs. Observer 1 | |
	Obs1	Obs2	Computed	Obs2	Computed	Obs2	Computed
1	122	109	186	13	76	11	62
2	170	199	148	35	36	21	21
3	104	128	107	26	15	25	14
4	146	162	145	18	23	12	16-
5	122	172	181	52	77	43	63
6	122	146	132	28	42	23	34
7	125	153	144	28	37	22	30
8	102	124	101	22	17	22	17
9	117	119	128	14	17	12	15
10	100	113	92	15	24	15	24
11	90	102	95	18	21	20	23
12	108	107	111	11	15	10	14
13	142	152	146	24	22	17	15
14	30	80	112	6	44	8	55
15	112	116	135	12	39	11	35
16	251	274	246	29	29	12	12
17	133	141	164	16	37	12	23
18	120	110	109	20	17	17	14
19	117	113	148	18	39	15	33
20	184	185	191	25	53	14	29
Mean	128.4	140.3	141.0	21.5	34.0	16.8	26.5
S.Dev.	37.0	42.5	37.5	9.9	17.8		

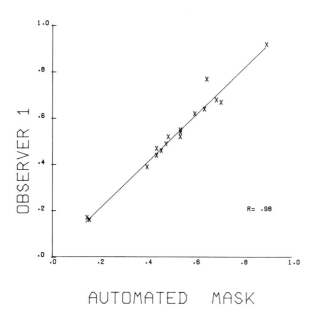

FIG. 5. Ejection fraction for automated masks vs. those drawn by Observer 1.

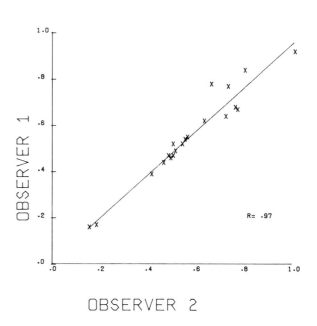

FIG. 6. Ejection fraction for masks
drawn by Observer 1 vs. those drawn
by Observer 2.

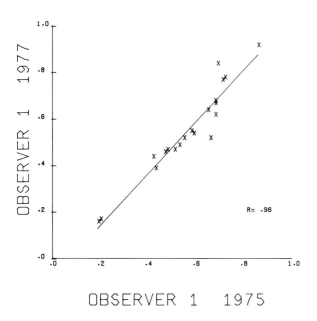

FIG. 7. Ejection fraction for masks
previously drawn by Observer 1 vs.
those recently drawn by Observer 1.

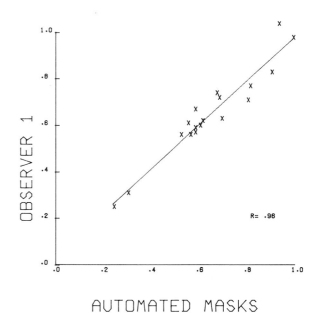

FIG. 8. Peak normalized ejection
rate for automated masks vs. those
drawn by Observer 1.

single observer over an extended period of time. Hence its accuracy is probably not less and reproducibility better than hand drawn masks.

REFERENCES

1. Green, M.V., Ostrow, H.G., Douglas, M.A., et al: High Temporal Resolution ECG-Gated Scintigraphic Angiocardiography. J Nucl Med 16:95-98 (1975).

2. Goris, M.L., Daspit, S.G., McLaughlin, P., Kriss, J.P.: Interpolative Background Subtraction. J Nucl Med 17:744-747 (1976).

3. Robinson, G.S.:Edge Detection by Compass Gradient Masks. Computer Graphics and Image Processing 6:492-501 (1977).

MULTIFACETED EVALUATION OF LEFT VENTRICULAR FUNCTION BY THE FIRST TRANSIT TECHNIQUE USING ANGER TYPE CAMERAS AND AN OPTIMIZED PROTOCOL: CORRELATION WITH BIPLANE ROENTGEN ANGIOGRAPHY.

Dan G. Pavel, M.D., Ernest Byrom, Ph.D., Bronte Ayres, M.D.,
Raymond J. Pietras, M.D., Jesus A. Bianco, M.D., Charles Kanakis, Jr., M.D.

Sections of Nuclear Medicine and Cardiology
University of Illinois Medical Center
Chicago, Illinois   60612

A computer macroprogram has been developed to optimize the processing of first transit radionuclide cardiac studies (RCS) from Anger type cameras and maximize the information obtained. To take into account the difference between the end-diastolic (ED) and end-systolic (ES) sizes of the normal heart, regions of interest (ROIs) are defined simultaneously and semiautomatically for both ED and ES. The free borders are defined by the isocount line that gives the best simultaneous fit on both images. A perisystolic horseshoe background ROI is used. For improved accuracy and reliability the valve plane is drawn simultaneously on the ED image and on a subtraction image, ED - ES, using a "double bug" technique. In addition to a value for Ejection Fraction (EF) and a left ventricular time-activity curve, the final product includes: cinematic and static displays of the 16-image composite cardiac cycle, a combined display of ED and ES images with their respective ROI outlines and the outlines superimposed, two subtraction images and a display of color-coded isocontours for the frames intermediate between ED and ES. This array of results allows also the evaluation of regional wall motion abnormalities and their functional consequences. On 40 consecutive patients, the results were compared with those from biplane roentgen angiography (BA). The correlation coefficient was 0.89. The mean values were for BA 52.4 and for RCS 54.4 which is not a statistically significant difference. Calculations were also made by the usual single ROI method which was found to underestimate EF significantly (mean: 46.5). In detecting regional wall motion abnormality, RCS agreed with BA in 34 of the 40 patients (85%); one case was falsely positive (2.5%) and 5 were falsely negative (12.5%). In conclusion, a wide array of accurate data can be obtained by this method on Anger type gamma cameras.

Radionuclide cardiac studies have gained acceptance today as noninvasive methods for the evaluation of left ventricular function. Among different approaches in use is the first-transit method which allows a functional evaluation of the left ventricle from data obtained during the first transit of a radionuclide bolus through the central circulation (5, 15, 17, 20). Originally this method led only to the calculation of ejection fraction (EF) and only recently have wall motion evaluations been attempted using older Anger type camera models (8). Multicrystal type cameras with built-in computers and a factory installed computer program have been used to obtain a wider variety of data with this method (6,14,18). We have decided to evaluate the possibilities of the Anger type cameras with this technique by developing a program which should optimize the data processing, take into account at least partially the spatial changes during a cardiac cycle, maximize the information obtained, and limit the intra-and interobserver variation.

MATERIALS AND METHODS

Data from forty consecutive patients (33 males, 7 females; age range 17-70, mean 47 years) having temporally comparable and technically suitable first-transit radionuclide cardiac studies and cardiac catheterizations were analyzed. The patients were catheterized to assess organic heart disease, chest pain or arrhythmias. Patients with significant mitral stenosis were not included.

The roentgen angiogram was a biplane technique* performed in 30° RAO and 60° LAO and the EF calculated by the area-length method of Dodge (3). The data were obtained from ventricular contractions originating from normal electrical depolarizations and none were preceded by extrasystoles.

The radionuclide study was performed on two different Anger type cameras: a standard size 1975 model,** and a large field of view 1977 model.*** The position was 30° RAO in 37 cases, and 1 case each in anterior, 55° LAO and 40° LPO. A bolus injection was given in an antecubital vein using a short polyethylene Jelco catheter, and a 15-20 cc saline flush, with manual pressure.

An Informatek Simis III computer was used. The acquisition was done in list mode onto hard disk, with maximum count rates of approximately 30-40 K/sec. Processing was under control of a user devised macroprogram. The principal display was a TV monitor refreshed by a 64K byte mode memory capable of simultaneous presentation of sixteen 64 x 64 matrix images or four 128 x 128 images in monochrome or color coding. Backup numerical data was displayed on a storage scope.

Processing begins with the selection of a rough left ventricular region of interest (ROI) on an image of the levophase, and the generation of a time activity curve from a sequence of 130 high frequency frames, a technique similar to those of earlier investigators (5, 18, 15, 17, 20). The duration of these frames is 30, 40 or 50 msec depending upon the patient's heart rate, in order for 16 frames to approximately fit the duration of one cardiac cycle. No frames longer than 50 msec are used even for slow heart rates,

---

* Philips Medical Systems, ** G.E. Portacamera, *** Searle Radiographics

which leads to the omission of the slow filling phase in such cases. After smoothing by a 9-point filter (13), this curve is displayed together with time-coordinates of maxima and minima, located by software. Peaks are selected primarily on the basis of consistency of the duration of the systole, secondarily on the duration of the complete cycle. Four to seven cardiac cycles are then summed and the composite cycle obtained is immediately available for endless loop movie format evaluation.

The next step generates a zoomed display from each of the 16 frames of the cardiac cycle. This is done by interpolating to a 64 x 64 matrix size the 32 x 32 region containing the left ventricle. Four 9-point spatial smoothings are applied, as well as a pairing of successive frames (time smoothing). This heavy smoothing is for purposes of display only.

The end-diastolic (ED) and end-systolic (ES) frames are now chosen from the 16 images and displayed in 128 x 128 size, with interpolation, on the TV monitor, in monochrome. The cardiac silhouette is then accentuated by varying TV contrast. Various isocontours, representing the same absolute count level in both images are generated iteratively and the best simultaneous fit to the ED and ES cardiac silhouettes is chosen (Fig. 1A).

A horseshoe background region is now generated around the ES outline two elements out and three wide, the operator assigning the limits only (Fig. 1B) in such a way that the horseshoe does not encompass areas of highly variable activity around the base of the ventricle. The counts per matrix element in this region, on the ES image, constitute the background correction, which is subtracted as a constant from all the 16 smoothed images.

At this point a new color display is generated containing the background corrected ED and ES together with the functional subtraction images ED - ES and ES - ED. The ED valve plane delineation is performed on this display using a double cursor (2) for simultaneous use of both ED and ED - ES images (Fig. 1C) to complete the ED ROI. The ES valve plane is then defined using alternately monochrome and color display for guidance, and arbitrarily superimposing the middle portion of the valve plane over the corresponding ED portion (Fig. 2B, 3B).

The next step deals with the EF computation and time-activity curve generation. The contents of the ROIs previously defined is taken from a set of matrices which have only undergone zooming and interpolation but not additional smoothing. Background correction is now done for ED and ES after normalization to their respective ROI sizes, and the ejection fraction is calculated:

$$EF = \frac{(ED\ cts - B1) - (ES\ cts - B2)}{ED\ cts - B1}$$

B1 = background normalized to ED ROI
B2 = background normalized to ES ROI

Sixteen point left ventricular activity (LVA) curves (C) are obtained for both ROIs after subtracting the corresponding constant background values (B1 and B2). A weighted interpolation yields the final C_{LVA}; its value at the n-th point is:

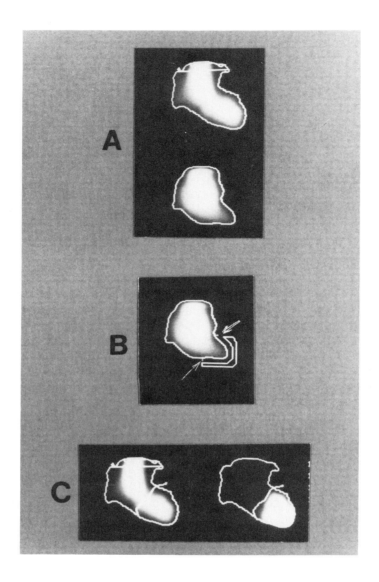

FIG. 1. (A) Best fit isocontours on ED and ES images. (B) For the background ROI, the operator indicates only two points on the ES contour (arrows). (C) A double cursor is used to define the valve plane. The same line is drawn simultaneously on both the ED image (left) and the difference image, ED − ES (right).

$$C_{LVA}(n) = \frac{(n-1)\ C_{ES}(n)\ +\ (a-n)\ C_{ED}(n)}{a-1}$$ where "a" = frame number at ES,

and C = curve. Thus $C_{LVA}(1) = C_{ED}(1)$ and $C_{LVA}(a) = C_{ES}(a)$.

The ejection fraction was also calculated by the usual method, in which both ES and ED counts are taken from the ED ROI, and the two background corrections are identical and normalized to the ED ROI size.

In four cases attempts were made to vary the free border contours by choosing them looser and then tighter by as much as 10% of the optimum contour, and in five cases the calculations were done by 3 different observers (D.P., E.B., B.A.) independently.

The end product of the processing consists of several composite color displays: the first represents the composite cardiac cycle (Fig. 2A, 3A). The second shows the ED and ES images with their respective ROI outlines, the ROI outlines superimposed, the ejection fraction value, and the time activity curves (Fig. 2B, 3B). The third contains the subtraction images ED - ES and ES - ED (Fig. 2C, 3C). The last display is generated by superimposing a series of color coded isocontours (of the same count value determined earlier as defining the free borders of the ventricle) from every second image intermediate between ED and ES (Fig. 2D, 3D).

The wall motion was evaluated in comparison with the corresponding biplane angiography (BA) image. The RAO was divided into 5 segments (anterior, anterolateral, apical, inferior, inferoposterior) according to the description of Schulze (16). For the case done in LAO only three segments were used (16). Only the presence or absence of abnormality was considered. Segment #5 in RAO (inferoposterior) was left out of the evaluation.

RESULTS

The forty values of ejection fraction obtained by BA and from the radionuclide study, using ED and ES ROIs, were compared. The correlation coefficient between the two sets of results was 0.89 (Fig. 4A). The mean of the BA results was 52.4, with values ranging from 23 to 83. The mean of the radionuclide results was 54.4 with a range from 19 to 79. Paired-t analysis indicates that the difference between the means is not statistically significant ($p > 0.05$). The BA values were also compared to the radionuclide study results using the ED ROI only. The correlation coefficient was 0.85 (Fig. 4B). The radionuclide method, using the ED ROI only, gave a mean ejection fraction of 46.5, with values ranging from 15 to 76. The underestimation in this case is statistically significant based on the paired-t analysis ($p < 0.001$).

In the four cases in which the free borders were deliberately changed, in order to test for possible inter- and intra-observer variations, the EF values came within 5% of the original calculated value. The results obtained by the 3 different observers were within ± 5% of their mean in each of the five cases.

Wall motion normality or abnormality was correctly predicted by the radionuclide study in 34 of the 40 patients (85%). There were five false negative results (12.5%) and one false positive (2.5%).

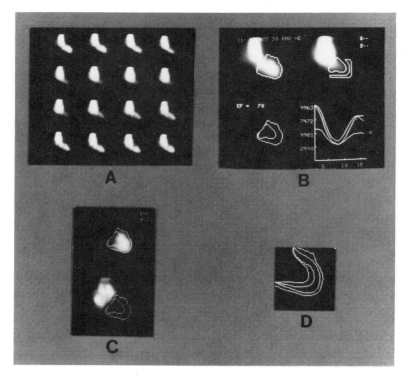

FIG. 2. Normal study. (A) Composite cardiac cycle; (B) ED and ES frames, superimposed ROI outlines, EF value, and time-activity curves (the middle one is the weighted interpolation between ED and ES curves); (C) subtraction images ED − ES (above) and ES − ED (below); (D) intermediate iso-contours.

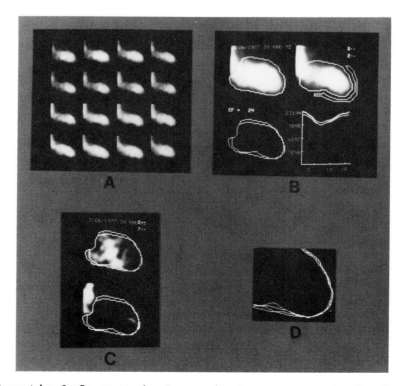

FIG. 3. Asymptomatic left ventricular apical aneurysm. A, B, C, D: same as Fig. 2.

DISCUSSION

The protocols and programs in use for first transit studies are quite varied due to the relative novelty of the technique, and to substantial differences in available equipment (5, 8, 14, 15, 17, 20). The results of this study indicate that it is possible to obtain a wide variety of data by using the most commonly available instrument, the Anger type camera. Even though its inherent dead time is greater than that of the multi-crystal devices, the newest models are quite satisfactory for first-transit studies when appropriate programs are available and when the computer displays are flexible enough.

The distinguishing feature of the protocol described is the assignment of separate ROIs to ED and ES in processing first transit studies. In all past publications one ROI was used, defined either on the ED frame or on a composite image of the whole cardiac cycle. From a theoretical point of view, this approach is a severe approximation, because of the spatial changes that occur during a cardiac cycle, and in practice we found a tendency to underestimate the EF when using it.* This tendency can be avoided to a certain extent by variations in the amount and type of background subtraction (15) but then the method becomes quite dependent upon the precision of the background ROI. In general when an ED ROI alone is used, the background corrections for both ED and ES counts are normalized to that ROI size, which overestimates ES background. This compensates to an unpredictable degree for the use of too large a ROI for ES. As no optimal background correction method seems to be presently at hand (10) we have adopted the approach that seems closest to physiological and anatomical reality, using the perisystolic area initially suggested by Parker (9) and the constant value subtraction (after normalization for ROI size) previously used for EKG-synchronized studies (4, 9). While the background activity certainly varies in time, this fluctuation can be considered minimal during the peak activity cycles of the levophase, as shown in earlier publications (17, 20).

The delineation of the valve planes has always been the most difficult part in this type of study. Three features of the program are designed to increase the accuracy and reproducibility of this step: the interpolative zooming improves the visualization of the whole left ventricular area; the display of the functional subtraction image (ED - ES) at this stage provides an objective guide to this part of the border; and, probably most important, the double cursor technique (2) allows the boundary to be traced simultaneously on both the anatomic ED image and the subtraction image (Fig. 1C). For the delineation of the valvular plane of the systolic image its central portion has been empirically set to overlap the diastolic border. While this is not physiologically accurate one should consider that even in roentgen angiography the valve plane setting in systole is not easy to determine and that there are different opinions about what should be included in it. Also, in that particular area the number of cts/pixel is usually smaller than in the mid ventricular area, and thus makes a smaller contribution to the calculation of EF by the net integral count method.

Intra- and interoperator variability is minimized by tying the selection of three ROIs together. Since the free borders of the ED and ES ROIs

---

* A similar tendency has been noted for EKG synchronized studies (1).

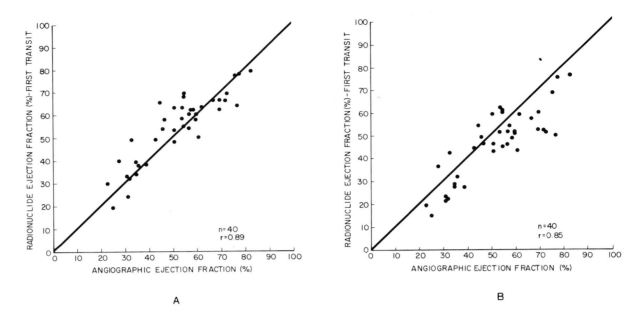

FIG. 4. Correlation between EF values from biplane angiography and radionuclide studies: (A) using ED and ES ROIs; (B) using only ED ROI.

are defined by isocontours of the same count value, and the background set
a fixed distance from the ES border, no ROI can be varied without changing
the others (Fig. 1). In addition the program guides the operator to a great
extent: once the isocount line has been chosen most of the free ventricular
borders in ED and ES are automatically assigned, and for the valve planes
the double cursor technique coupled with the use of the subtraction image
makes the operation much more reliable even though not entirely operator
independent. The reproducibility has proven very satisfactory even when
deliberate attempts have been made to loosen or tighten the isocount values
by ± 10%: not more than 5% variation was introduced.

The time-activity curves generated from the two ROIs are strikingly
different (Fig. 2B). It is apparent that each of them can be considered
valid only in one point: the origin of the ED curve (upper one) because its
ROI corresponds to the ED projection, and the minimum of the ES curve (lower
one) because its ROI corresponds to the ES projection. Since emphasis is
now being placed on time-activity curves for the evaluation of ventricular
function (7), we have attempted to obtain a more accurate representation of
the whole curve by the weighted interpolation. This appears to be the only
alternative presently available for a more accurate curve, short of establishing multiple ROIs instead of two. While the latter has been done automatically by computer in EKG-synchronized studies in the LAO view (12), it
does not seem possible at the present time for the first transit study in
RAO. If the EF calculations were done only on the curve originating from
the ED ROI the reason for a systematic underestimation is evident (Fig. 2B).

For correlation we have used biplane roentgen angiography (BA) considered the most reliable reference today especially in abnormal left ventricles

(19). While the correlation coefficient is very good (Fig. 4A), of even more importance is the fact that there is no significant difference between the means and thus no significant tendency to under or overestimation. When the single ROI method is used, while the correlation coefficient is still good (Fig. 4B), the mean indicates a statistically significant underestimation.

The presence or absence of wall motion abnormalities was correctly predicted in 85% of the cases by combining the evaluation of the endless loop movie format, the superimposed ED and ES outlines, the functional subtraction images and the color coded isocontour displays of intermediate frames. The evaluation of the posteroinferior segment (#5) on RAO views is unreliable due to adjacent structures, difficult delineation of the ES border and minimal contribution to the stroke volume. Overall the multiplicity of displays appeared to be an excellent adjunct for improved diagnostic accuracy in borderline cases. The striking differences between a normal and abnormal ventricle are clearly seen in Figs. 2 and 3. When there is marked abnormality (extensive akinesis or dyskinesis) the reverse subtraction image ES - ED elicits positive areas indicating precisely the most affected area.

Practically all the data obtained with the protocol described can be condensed on 4 color polaroids, by taking advantage of the display flexibility available on our system (11). These images can be attached to the final report which simplifies the filing and eases the comparison with follow-up studies.

In conclusion, an array of useful and reliable information, more extensive than any previously reported for work on Anger type cameras, can be obtained from first transit radionuclide studies. In view of the known convenience of the method, which does not require simultaneous ECG recording and involves minimal patient and camera time, these results indicate a great potential for expanded use of the first transit technique.

Acknowledgement: We are grateful for the assistance of A. Purohit, Ph.D. in the statistical analysis of the results.

REFERENCES

1. Borer JS, Bacharach SL, Green MV, et al: Real-time radionuclide cine-angiography in the noninvasive evaluation of global and regional left ventricular function at rest and during exercise in patients with coronary artery disease. N Eng J Med 296:839-844, 1977.

2. Byrom E, Pavel DG: Improved computer definition of regions of interest by using a double "bug" method. (submitted for publication).

3. Dodge HT, Sandler H, Baxley WA, et al: Usefulness and limitations of radiographic methods for determining left ventricular volume. Amer J Cardiol 18:10-18, 1966.

4. Green MV, Ostrow HG, Douglas MA, et al: High temporal resolution ECG-gated scintigraphic angiocardiography. J Nucl Med 16:95-98, 1975.

5. Hamilton GW, Weaver WD, Williams DG, et al: Calculation of ejection fraction from first transit radionuclide data: A comparison of several methods with contrast angiography. (abstr) J Nucl Med 17:556, 1976.

6.   Jones RH, Scholz PM: Data enhancement techniques for radionuclide cardiac studies. [In] Medical Radionuclide Imaging, IAEA, Vienna 2:255-266, 1977.

7.   Marshall RC, Freedman GS, Berger J, et al: Left ventricular contractility as assessed by normalized ejection velocity utilizing quantitative radionuclide angiocardiography and a computerized multi-crystal scintillation camera. (abstr) J Nucl Med 17:556, 1976.

8.   Myers RW: Single transit non-gated radionuclide angiocardiography for assessing left ventricular wall motion and ejection fraction. Clin Nucl Med 1:191-197, 1976.

9.   Parker JA, Secker-Walker R, Hill R, et al: A new technique for the calculation of left ventricular ejection fraction. J Nucl Med 13:649-651,1972.

10.   Pierson RN, Alan S, Kemp HG, et al: Radiocardiography in clinical cardiology. Sem Nucl Med 7:85-100, 1977.

11.   Pavel DG, Byrom E, Bianco JA: A method for increasing the accuracy of the ejection fraction and left ventricular volume curve. (abstr) J Nucl Med 18:641, 1977.

12.   Pitt B, Strauss HW: Evaluation of ventricular function by radioisotopic techniques. N Engl J Med 296:1097-1099, 1977.

13.   Savitsky A, Golay MJE: Smoothing and differentiation by simplified least square procedures. Analytical Chemistry 36:1627, 1964.

14.   Schad N: Nontraumatic assessment of left ventricular wall motion and regional stroke volume after myocardial infarction. J Nucl Med 18:333-341,1977.

15.   Schelbert HR, Verba HW, Johnson AD, et al: Nontraumatic determination of left ventricular ejection fraction by radionuclide angiocardiography. Circulation 51:902, 1975.

16.   Schulze RA, Humphries JO, Griffith LSC: Left ventricular and coronary angiographic anatomy. Circulation 55:839-843, 1977.

17.   Van Dyke D, Anger HO, Sullivan RW, et al: Cardiac evaluation from radioisotope dynamics. J Nucl Med 13:585-592, 1972.

18.   Van Hove ED, Heck LL, Kight JL: Improved myocardial infarct localization by combination of scintigraphy and ventricular wall motion evaluation. Radiology 124:425-429, 1977.

19.   Vogel JHK, Cornish D, McFadden RB: Underestimation of ejection fraction with single plane angiography in coronary artery disease. Chest 64:217-221, 1973.

20.   Weber PM, dos Remedios LV, Jaske IA: Quantitative radioisotopic angiocardiography. J Nucl Med 13:815-822, 1972.

NON-INTERACTIVE IDENTIFICATION OF THE LEFT VENTRICULAR AREA

Michael L. Goris, M.D., Ph.D.
Stanford University School of Medicine
Stanford, CA 94305

ABSTRACT

The definition of the left ventricular region on functional criteria has been described. There are two factors which complicate this approach: not all extraventricular points have zero values for the parameters measured nor are they homogeneous within the ventricular region. Those problems additionally decrease the ease by which parametric images can be represented and interpreted, e.g., a zero D-S difference has a different meaning within or without the left ventricular region of interest. A method is presented and discussed by which the left ventricular region of interest is determined using parameters reflecting ventricular changes of activity, as well as their statistical significance level and their distribution over levels of activity in the end-diastolic image.

INTRODUCTION

Most described methods for the determination of regions of interest over the left ventricle are based on operator intervention and pattern recognition (1,2,3). The precision of this determination is not critical, except for the degree by which the outflow tract is included (4). Yet, the precise recognition method used to identify the valvular plane is not mentioned (4) or is assumed to be trivial (5). None of the methods actually used for the selection has been described in a form which appears suitable for automation. The actual role of edge detection algorithms (6,7) needs further exploration.

In the book: Quantitative Nuclear Cardiography (8) Pierson and Van Dyke mention a method originally used by Kriss: the region of interest is identified as the region with a positive count difference between the cumulative end-diastolic and end-systolic images (5).

Pattern recognition is still heavily relied on. Firstly, random error produces non-zero values for the difference even in non-ventricular (background) regions. Secondly, in cases with akinesia or dyskinesia, regions with zero difference have to be included. The valvular plane, however, is usually easily identified by this method, since it appears as a linear demarcation between zero and non-zero differences, in a region with high counts in the end-diastolic image.

RATIONALE

Given a set of images representing activity distribution at subsequent times during the systolic cycle, the following can be postulated:

1. Significant decrease in count rates between end-diastolic and end-systole will be clustered in the left ventricular region. Additionally, significant variation in count rate during the whole systolic cycle will be clustered in the major vessel region.

2. In regions containing activity levels lower than the ventricular or large vessel regions, decrease of count rate and count-rate variations which appear significant are less likely to occur. Hence, a distribution function of significant decrease and variation as a function of count rates in the end-diastolic image will show a demarcation at the threshold level below which no ventricular or large vessel activity was detected.

3. Conversely, occasional significant decrease or variation in regions with less than threshold count rates in the end-diastolic image can be disregarded.

4. In the majority of cases dyskinesia or akinesia is proximal (closer to the apex) than the valvular plane. Hence, points with larger than threshold value in the end-diastolic image and which are proximal to the valvular plane should be included in the left ventricular region of interest if they are connected to it, even if no significant decrease was detected at this point.

To the extent that the four assumptions hold, the problem is trivial. Care is taken to document the final result in such a way that failure is easily recognized. In those cases operator intervention can be requested at any step.

METHOD BY STEPS

Step 1. From a set of chronological images, the end-diastolic and end-systolic images are easily identified, by computing positive differences between the images by sets of two.

Step 2. For each point in the projection matrix a regression analysis is carried through for all the frames between end-diastole and end-systole. Significant negative slopes are mapped in a slope image. The level of significance to be set is dependent on the type of preprocessing (smoothing) but does not vary from one case to another, given a constant preprocessing method.

Step 3. In the same way count-rate variation is computed on a point-by-point basis for all the frames of the systolic cycle (diastole to diastole) and a significant (versus Poisson statistics) variation map is constructed.

Step 4. Two distribution functions are constructed, for the slope and variation map, respectively. The independent variable of those distribution functions is the count rate in the end-diastolic image; the dependent variable is the sum of the magnitudes of slopes and variation, respectively. For each of those distribution functions, a threshold is determined by fitting a line at the point of maximum increase and determining the intercept with the X-axis. The mean of the two intercept values is used as the threshold level of count rates. (Fig. 1)

Step 5. The threshold value is subtracted from the end-diastolic image count rates. Negative results are set equal to zero. All points which are zero in the end-diastolic map are also set to zero in the slope map. Since the slope itself is independent of background, since it is computed in a linear regression of the type bx+a, no further correction for size is necessary. (Fig. 2A, 2B)

Step 6. Small clusters of positive slope values remaining at this time are further eliminated. The result is very much independent from the clustering strategy used, as long as the size of the area and the size of the slope values are used concurrently as criteria. Following this a normalized slope image is produced in which only left ventricular regions are allowed to have non-zero values. (Fig. 2C, 2D)

Step 7. Two binary images are now framed, one in which non-zero value in the corrected end-diastolic image is set to 1, and the same for the final (corrected and unclustered) slope map. On those images a center of gravity is determined for the non-zero value. It is assumed that the center of gravity in the binary end-diastolic image is distal (towards the aorta) from the one in the binary slope image.

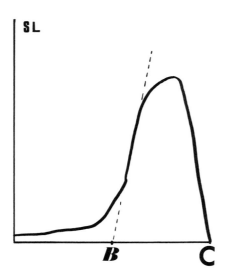

FIG. 1. Density distribution of slope values (SL) as a function of counts in the end-diastolic image (C). The dotted line is computed by linear regression at the point of maximum slope. The value of C at the intercept B is assumed to be the threshold value.

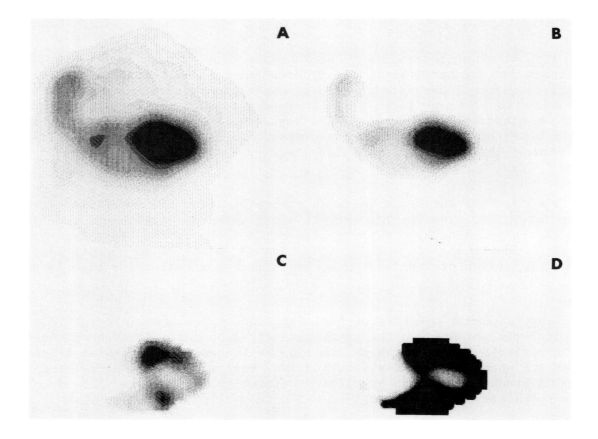

FIG. 2. Data processing. In (A) the original end-diastolic image is shown. The result following background subtraction is shown in (B). Values for the slope, exclusive of regions below background level, are shown in (C). Normalizing the slope to the net end-diastolic value results in (D).

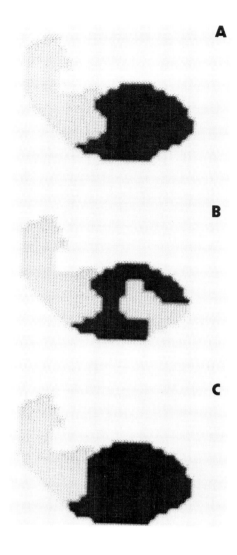

FIG. 3. Determination of the region of interest:
(A) and (B) represent the binary representation
of positive points in the end-diastolic image
(gray) and positive points in the slope image.
In case (B), a section of the ventricle is akinetic. The region of interest should include all
of the dark in (A) and (B), but more than it in
(B). Using the logic described in the text, the
selected region is represented as black in (C),
for both cases.

Step 8. The region of interest is now determined by scanning the two
binary images from two orthogonal directions, such that in each direction
the coordinate of the center of gravity in the binary end-diastolic image
is smaller than the coordinate of the center of gravity in the binary slope
image.

A point is included in the region of interest if, and only if, it has
a non-zero value in the binary end-diastolic image, and itself, or a preceding
point on the scanning line, has a non-zero value in the binary slope image.
(Fig. 3)

DISCUSSION

Ideally one would identify regions of interest exclusively by functional
criteria. However, since the target organ may fail in part to exhibit its
natural (normal) functional behavior, additional criteria should be used.
Furthermore, with noisy data sets, as are usually available in nuclear medi-

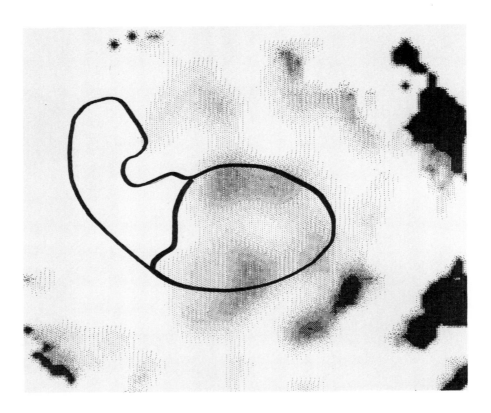

FIG. 4. In this image the slope value has been normalized by the original
end-diastolic values, while non-zero values in background regions were not
eliminated. The resulting image is unclear and lacks the definition of
Fig. 2D.

cine, one needs to guard against count-rate behaviors which mimic organ
function, outside of the organ's projection area.

The first step to define the region of interest is the determination of
a threshold, below which no target activity will be found. There really is
no rational way to determine this threshold as a function of maximum count
rate, a much favored approach in general (9). Determining the background from
surrounding areas (5,8,10) assumes that the region of interest is already
recognized. Functional criteria can be used, however, in a wide range of
cases. One should emphasize, however, that this allows one to determine
average size, but not shape, of the background (10,11).

One of the advantages of eliminating background lies in the clarity
of the parametric images which otherwise contain too much irrelevant information (11). But mainly the simplified images allow one to use simple logic
for the inclusion of non-functional target areas in the region of interest.
(Fig. 4)

REFERENCES

1. Schelbert HR, Verba JW, Johnson AD, et al: Non-traumatic determination of left ventricular ejection fraction by radionuclide angiocardiography. Circulation 51: 902-909, 1975.

2. Berman DS, Salel AS, De Nardo GL, et al: Clinical assessment of left ventricular regional contraction patterns and ejection fraction by high resolution gated scintigraphy. J Nucl Med 16: 865-874, 1975.

3. Strauss WH, Zaret BL, Hurley PJ, et al: A scintigraphic method for measuring left ventricular ejection fraction in man without cardiac catheterization. The Am J of Card 28: 575-580, 1971.

4. Marshall RC, Berger, JH, Costin JC, et al: Assessment of cardiac performance with quantitative radionuclide angiocardiography. Circulation 56: 820-829, 1977.

5. Myers RW: Single transit non-gated radionuclide angiocardiography for assessing left ventricular wall motion and ejection fraction. Clin Nucl Med 1: 191-197, 1976.

6. Cahill P, Ho L, Ornstein E, et al: Operator independent edge detection algorithms in nuclear medicine. J Nucl Med 18: 607, 1977.

7. Burrow R, Pond M, Rehn T, et al: A semi-automatic edge detection program for the analysis of multiple gated acquisition cardiac blood pool images. J Nucl Med 18: 608, 1977.

8. Pierson RN, Van Dyke DC: Analysis of left ventricular function. Quantitative Nuclear Cardiography (Ed: Pierson, Kriss, Jones, MacIntyre), p. 123-154. John Wiley & Sons publishers, 1975.

9. Narahara KA, Hamilton GW, Williams DL, et al: Myocardial imaging with thallium-201: an experimental model for analysis of true myocardial and background image components. J Nucl Med 18: 781-786, 1977.

10. Goris ML, Daspit SG, McLaughlin P, et al: Interpolative background subtraction. J Nucl Med 17: 744-747, 1976.

11. Geffers H, Adam WE, Kampmann H, et al: Data processing and functional imaging in radionuclide ventriculography. Presented at the Vth International Conference on "Information Processing in Medical Imaging," Nashville, TN, June 1977.

MYOCARDIAL WALL EVALUATION
WITH THALLIUM-201
MULTIPLE GATED ACQUISITION

Jaroslaw Muz, Steven J. Figiel,
and Thomas M. Kumpuris

Harper Division
Harper-Grace Hospitals
Radiology Department
Nuclear Medicine Section
Detroit, Michigan 48201

ABSTRACT

Fifty-four patients underwent evaluation of myocardium utilizing Thallium-201 and the multiple gated acquisition (MUGA) program. Static and MUGA images were obtained simultaneously. Static, systolic and diastolic images were evaluated separately. Thirty-eight patients demonstrated perfusion defects. Of these thirty-eight patients, twelve showed myocardial perfusion abnormalities, detected with the MUGA program only. Blurring of images due to cardiac wall motion can be eliminated by separating systolic from diastolic images. Evaluation of separated diastolic images is the most important factor in detection of small myocardial perfusion defects.

INTRODUCTION

Thallium-201 myocardial perfusion examination has become an accepted modality in detecting the presence of myocardial ischemia or infarction (1-3).

Thallium-201 (Tl-201) is a cyclotron produced radionuclide with useful energy from 69 to 80 keV. Its physical half-life is 73 hours. When injected intravenously in the form of thallous chloride, it demonstrates biological characteristics similar to those of potassium (4,5). It is extracted from the blood compartment, particularly by myocardium, and is transported through the sodium-potassium pump intracellularly. The distribution of Tl-201 through the myocardium depends on the status of the coronary arteries. Areas of diminished myocardial blood flow will result in locally diminished Tl-201 transport and will appear as "cold spots" on the myocardial scintigrams.

Tl-201 imaging is most frequently used for non-invasive evaluation of regional myocardial perfusion (6). Since the myocardium normally moves during contractions, images obtained with a scintillation camera are blurred due to motion effect (7). As a result of blurring, the chamber of the left ventricle appears to be disproportionately small and the myocardium thick with ill-defined edges. This deteriorates the diagnostic quality of a myocardial image to the extent that small underperfused regions can escape detection. In order to eliminate myocardial motion effect, we apply the multiple gated acquisition (MUGA) computer technique. MUGA allows us to acquire data for subsequent left myocardial wall motion display and separate systolic from diastolic images for detailed analysis.

MATERIALS AND METHODS

Patients
Fifty-four patients underwent Tl-201 myocardial perfusion evaluation utilizing a gamma camera and the MUGA computer program. Of these 54 patients, 24 had a resting examination. (Table 1A) The average age of this group of patients was 59 years, ranging from 31 to 85 years. All patients had electrocardiographic (ECG) changes, 13 had myocardial infarction (MI). Six patients had cardiac catheterization; five of them demonstrated coronary artery abnormalities.

Thirty patients had exercise Tl-201 examinations. (Table 1B) The average age of this group was 49 years, ranging from 26 to 68 years. Ten patients had normal ECG's, six had MI, two had left bundle branch block, one had right bundle branch block, eight had nonspecific ST-T changes and three had arrhythmia. Ten patients had cardiac catheterization; nine of them demonstrated coronary artery changes. The exercise test was positive in five patients, negative in eleven and inconclusive in fourteen.

Radionuclide imaging
Resting studies: With the patient in the upright position, and fasting if possible, 1.5-2.0 mCi of Tl-201 (thallous chloride) is administered intravenously. Imaging is initiated ten minutes after injection. Static images are obtained in anterior (ANT), left anterior oblique (LAO) and left lateral (LLAT) projections. Five hundred thousand counts are acquired for each static image. At the same time, data are acquired using the MUGA computer

program. Forty thousand counts are acquired per frame for twenty-eight
frames per view for myocardial wall imaging. The average time for MUGA
acquisition is 25.2 minutes for each view, depending on the administered
dose, status of imaged myocardium and patient's size.

Exercise studies: The patient is exercised to the point of tolerance on
on the treadmill in the Exercise Laboratory. At the peak of exercise,
1.5-2.0 mCi of Tl-201 is injected intravenously with continuation of exercise for thirty to sixty seconds past peak. Within four minutes after the
injection, precordial imaging is initiated in LAO projection utilizing a
portable scintillation camera. Three hundred thousand counts are acquired
for a static image. On completion of the LAO view in the Exercise Laboratory,
all patients are immediately transferred to the Nuclear Medicine Department
for simultaneous static and MUGA image acquisition. Five hundred thousand
counts are acquired per each static view. Forty thousand counts are acquired
per frame for twenty-eight frames per view with the MUGA program. The acquisition time averages 25.2 minutes per view. The shortest acquisition time
was eleven minutes per view; the longest forty-six minutes per view.

Instrumentation
Immediate post-exercise studies were obtained utilizing an Ohio-Nuclear
Sigma 420 portable scintillation camera with a low-energy high-resolution
collimator.

Resting, post-exercise and delayed studies were performed on either a Searle
LFOV or an Ohio-Nuclear 410 scintillation camera. Low-energy all-purpose
collimators were used with both instruments. Both cameras were interfaced
with the Medical Data Systems (MDS) trinary computer with the capability of
multiple gated acquisition - MUGA and MUGX programs.

A Brattle Instrument Corporation physiological synchronizer was used as a
gate instrument.

Data Processing
The acquired data can be displayed in movie mode and/or systole-diastole
mode. We routinely use systole-diastole mode. It takes approximately five
minutes to process data in this mode.

RESULTS

Static and MUGA Tl-201 images were obtained simultaneously in fifty-four
patients. All static images were obtained in three standard projections. In
forty-two patients, MUGA images were obtained in three views. Eight patients
were examined in two projections and four in one projection.

Static and MUGA images were correlated with electrocardiograms (ECG), stress
tests and cardiac catheterization results. ECG changes of myocardial infarct (MI) and positive coronary arteriograms were accepted as the criteria
of myocardial lesion. Only sixteen patients had cardiac catheterization.
This makes the exact classification of this data very difficult.

In the resting group, static images were normal in two patients, whereas
MUGA images and coronary angiograms were positive. One patient had MI and
another nonspecific ST-T changes. We consider these two patients as

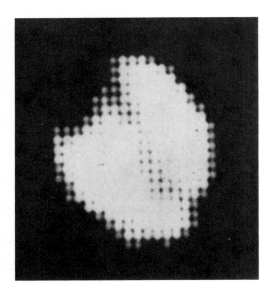 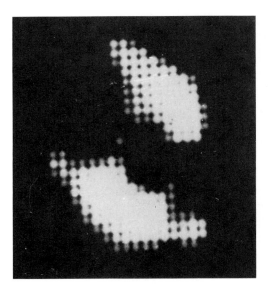

FIG. 1. (Left) Systolic image, ANT view of 35-year-old WF, diabetic with previous MI Jan. 77. This image was obtained from a computer oscilloscope after Tl-201 myocardial perfusion MUGA processing. This image revealed no apparent abnormality. (Right) Diastolic image, ANT view of the same patient revealed a perfusion defect in the anterolateral wall and apical region of the left ventricle.

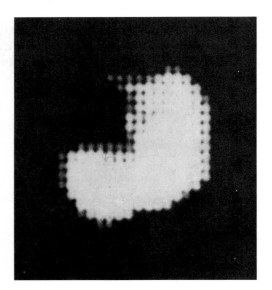 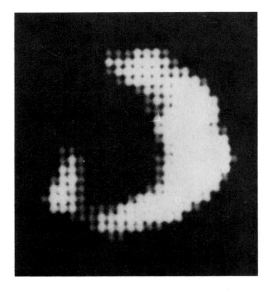

FIG. 2. (Left) Systolic Tl-201 myocardial perfusion image, LAO view of 47-year-old WM with MI and aortocoronary bypass. Systolic image is inconclusive. (Right) Diastolic image, LAO view of the same patient revealed markedly decreased perfusion to the septum.

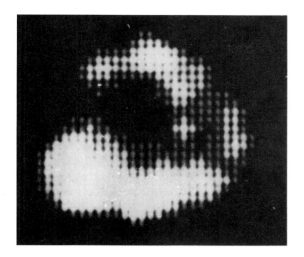 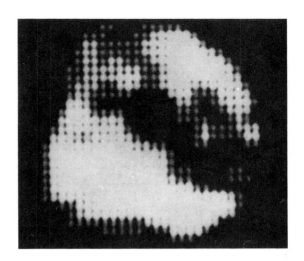

FIG. 3. (Left) Systolic image, ANT view of 40-year-old WM with MI and aorto-coronary bypass. Tl-201 MUGA image revealed an underperfused area in the anterolateral wall and apical region of the left ventricle. (Right) Diastolic image, ANT of the same patient revealed markedly decreased perfusion to the apex and anterolateral wall of the left ventricle.

TABLE 1.	A. RESTING Tl-201 Myocardial Perfusion Static vs MUGA Studies		B. EXERCISE Tl-201 Myocardial Perfusion Static vs MUGA Studies	
	Static Images	MUGA Images	Static Images	MUGA Images
No. of Patients	24	24	30	30
Normal perfusion	10	7	18	10
Perfusion defects	14	18	12	20
Perfusion defects – static only	0		0	
Perfusion defects – MUGA only		4		8

false negative for static imaging.

In the exercise group, there were six cases of false negative for static imaging.

In one case, MUGA study showed underperfused septum. Static images, ECG and stress tests were negative. We consider this case as a false positive for MUGA imaging.

In three cases, MUGA studies revealed double perfusion defects, whereas static studies revealed single defects. In seven cases, MUGA perfusion defects were more prominent as compared to static studies. In four cases, immediate post-exercise static studies were negative, whereas delayed static studies and MUGA studies were positive. All these patients had documented MI and positive coronary arteriograms. Two of these patients had coronary bypass.

DISCUSSION

Our studies showed that twelve of fifty-four patients demonstrated perfusion defects on MUGA studies which were not present on static images. (Table 2)

In four cases with documented myocardial damage (see results), immediate post-exercise static studies were negative, whereas delayed static and MUGA studies showed perfusion defects. This phenomenon is caused by blurring of images due to amplified wall motion of the post-exercise beating heart. Application of the MUGA program allows us to eliminate wall motion effect by separating systolic from diastolic images. In our opinion, the evaluation of separated diastolic images is the most important factor in detection of small myocardial perfusion defects.

Our study indicates that the MUGA program is a valuable adjunct for detection of Thallium-201 myocardial perfusion abnormalities.

There are, however, disadvantages to this program:
1. The acquisition time of twenty-five minutes is impractical for routine studies.
2. Transient myocardial ischemia could be difficult or impossible to detect with prolonged acquisition time per view. Reperfusion can occur during data acquisition of the first view.

TABLE 2.   Tl-201 Myocardial Perfusion
            Static vs MUGA Studies

	Static Images	MUGA Images
No. of Patients	54	54
Normal perfusion	28	16
Perfusion defects	26	38
Perfusion defects - static only	0	
Perfusion defects - MUGA only		12

REFERENCES

1. Pitt B, Strauss HW: Cardiovascular Nuclear Medicine. Semin Nucl Med
    7: 3-6, 1977

2. Pitt B, Strauss HW: Myocardial imaging in the non-invasive evaluation
    of patients with suspected ischemic heart disease. Am J Cardiol 37:
    797-806, 1976

3. Lenaers A, Block P, vanThiel E, et al: Segmental analysis of Tl-201
    stress myocardial scintigraphy. J Nucl Med 18: 509-516, 1977

4. Poe ND: Rationale and radiopharmaceuticals for myocardial imaging.
    Semin Nucl Med 7: 7-14, 1977

5. Lebowitz E, Greene, MW, Fairchild R, et al: Thallium-201 for medical
    use. 1. J Nucl Med 16: 151-155, 1975

6. Strauss HW, Holman L: Nuclear Cardiology. Course 409, page 3. RSNA
    Syllabus, Nuclear Medicine, 1977

7. Cook DJ, Bailey I, Strauss HW, et al: Thallium-201 for myocardial
    imaging: Appearance of the normal heart. J. Nucl Med 17: 583-589, 1976

IMAGE PROCESSING TECHNIQUES FOR THE EVALUATION

OF 201-THALLIUM MYOCARDIAL DISTRIBUTION

Michael J. Flynn, Ph.D.
Stephen N. Wiener, M.D.
Rachel M. Floyd, B.A.

Department of Radiology
The Mt. Sinai Hospital of Cleveland
University Circle
Cleveland, Ohio   44106

ABSTRACT

Factors which constrain 201-thallium myocardial image quality are considered and image processing methods suggested which minimize their influence on the final image. An algorithm which specifies a spatially variant background signal in the region of the myocardium is presented for which the estimate of the background signal is a weighted average of the pixel values along a predefined rectangular boundary surrounding the heart. An image smoothing algorithm is described which is a two-dimensional implementation of a one-dimensional technique described by Wertheim   for which the smoothing filter in frequency space is derived from the instrument resolution function. Finally, the blurring produced by myocardial wall motion is estimated and a method to eliminate motion blurring described. The net effect of background subtraction, image smoothing, and the elimination of motion degradation on 201-thallium myocardial images is described.

INTRODUCTION

Myocardial imaging with 201-thallium chloride challenges the performance capability of contemporary scintillation cameras. Reasons include the small dimensions of the myocardium, cardiac motion during the prolonged exposure interval, the low energy of the photons emitted by 201-thallium, the poor target to non-target ratio observed when the examination is performed at rest, and the presence of significant background activity in the vascular structures surrounding and within the heart. Nonetheless, the clinical benefits that may be derived from the examination in the management of patients with coronary artery disease have stimulated widespread utilization of the examination and provides strong motivation to optimize the image recording process. This paper considers those factors which constrain 201-thallium myocardial image quality and presents image processing methods to minimize their influence on the final image.

It has been previously demonstrated that a scintillation camera with good spatial and energy resolution is required for the evaluation of 201-thallium myocardial distribution (1,2). In addition, the video display of digitally stored information provides an improved presentation by standardizing the image gray levels and permitting quantitative evaluation of decreased uptake. The evaluation of 201-thallium myocardial distribution may be further improved by the implementation of image processing techniques which are specifically designed for 201-thallium myocardial images. Algorithms for background subtraction, image smoothing, and motion correction are considered below.

BACKGROUND SUBTRACTION

The need for background subtraction with myocardial images has been recognized for 201-thallium as well as for other myocardial radiopharmaceuticals. However, the actual characteristics of the background signal in 201-thallium myocardial images are poorly represented by a constant background level. Goris et al (3) have described an algorithm for interpolative background subtraction which specifies the background as a function of the activity surrounding the myocardium. An undesirable feature of the algorithm is an increase in the noise of the myocardial uptake signal since the background values are each determined from a small number of pixels. Narahara et al (4) have challenged the Goris algorithm and suggest the use of a constant 20% background signal. The experimental dog studies used to support their hypothesis do not, however, acknowledge the presence of a background signal originating from the blood pool in the chambers and large vessels of the heart. Furthermore, the variation in myocardial uptake between stress and non-stress examinations may not be accommodated by the simple specification of a background subtraction level. In the absence of a more definitive specification of the true background signal for 201-thallium images, we believe that optimal results may be achieved by examining the image signal level peripheral to the myocardium.

An algorithm which specifies a spatially-variant background signal in the region of the myocardium has been developed and implemented. The estimate of the background signal for each pixel is a weighted average of the pixel values along a predefined rectangular boundary surrounding the heart (see Figure 1). The weighting function utilized is equal to the inverse of the distance from the pixel for which the background is being estimated to the peripheral boundary pixel. The background estimate is thus analogous to the determination of the electric field within a specified charge boundary.

The spatially variant background signal determined from this algorithm is illustrated in Figure 2. The background estimate accommodates a subtle gradient, insensitive to localized hot or cold regions along the peripheral boundary. Since the algorithm utilizes all of the peripheral pixels for each estimate of the background signal, there is little statistical fluctuation in the background estimate. The magnitude of the background estimate at the center of the rectangular field of interest ranges from 30% to 48% as determined from the anterior view of ten randomly selected cases which included both stress and non-stress examinations. The algorithm additionally accomplishes a "coning" effect by zeroing all image cells outside the zone of the myocardium. This insures that the image gray scale is scaled to the maximum value observed in the myocardium. The algorithm has been implemented in Fortran and requires approximately nine minutes per image to execute on a PDP-11/40 computer with KE11-F floating instruction set.

IMAGE SMOOTHING

Because of the usually limited statistical information available in 201-thallium myocardial images along with the systematic appearance of both the normal myocardial distribution and the regions of defective distribution, the image is amenable to improved display by image smoothing. A wide variety of scintillation image smoothing techniques have been published in the literature of the last ten years. Most approaches use linear smoothing algorithms (5 - 10), many of which are applied in the frequency domain by using the fast fourier transformation (7 - 10); although, more recently, a number of non-linear and/or non-stationary smoothing algorithms have been presented (11 - 15). The basis for linear smoothing techniques is that noise frequencies adjacent to the spectrum of the image signal will suppress recognition (16) and thus the selective removal of high frequency components in an image (17) can enhance lesion detectability as long as "noise blobs" are not introduced which might be interpreted as false positive lesions (18). For the smoothing of 201-thallium images, we have employed a linear algorithm implemented in frequency space with a filter optimized for the measured thallium resolution characteristics of our imaging system.

The smoothing algorithm employed is a two-dimensional implementation of a one-dimensional technique described by Wertheim for which the smoothing filter in frequency space is derived from the instrument resolution function (19). The filter function, which is obtained from an analysis of the Van Cittert iterative deconvolution process, accomplishes low-pass filtering with no frequency enhancement (i.e., no image restoration). This function is given by the expression:

$$G_n(w) = 1 - \left[1 - G(w)\right]^n$$

where $G(w)$ is the Fourier transform of the instrument resolution function

SPATIALLY VARIANT BACKGROUND SUBTRACTION

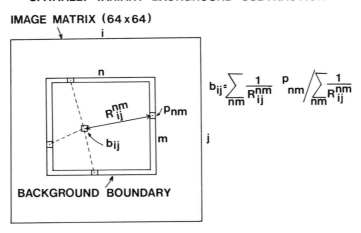

$$b_{ij} = \sum_{nm} \frac{1}{R_{ij}^{nm}} \; p_{nm} \bigg/ \sum_{nm} \frac{1}{R_{ij}^{nm}}$$

FIG. 1. The spatially variant background signal is a weighted average of the pixel values along a predefined rectangular boundary. The weighting function is equal to the inverse of the distance from the background pixel to each peripheral pixel.

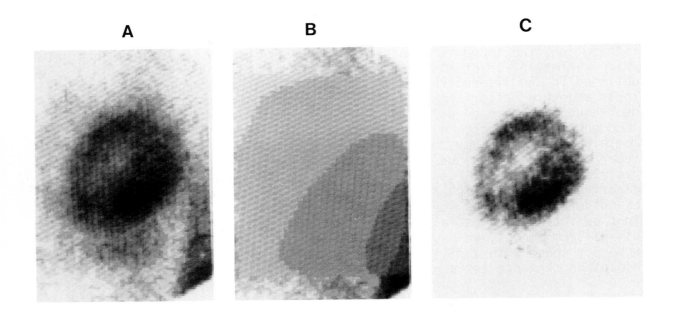

FIG. 2. Spatially variant background subtraction is illustrated by (A) the unprocessed image data from the LAO projection, (B) the spatially variant background signal estimated from A, and (C) the myocardial image after background subtraction.

(point spread function). The choice of n for smoothing a particular set
of data depends on the signal to noise ratio (19). For n equals 1, the
smoothing is accomplished with the resolution function itself. For a
signal of unknown shape hidden in white noise, n equals 1 optimizes the
signal to noise ratio but produces a loss of resolution. For n greater
than or equal to three, there is no appreciable loss of resolution (19).

The two-dimensional implementation of Wertheim's technique requires the
two-dimensional transform of the instrument's point spread function. We
have assumed that the point spread function is rotationally symmetric,
in which case its transform in a polar coordinate system, $G(w_r)$, is also
rotationally symmetric and equal to the one-dimensional transform of the
line spread function (20). This may easily be proven using the projection
theorem now employed for image reconstruction (21,22).

The filter function for this work has been derived from estimates of
the 201-thallium line spread function. These spread functions were
measured by placing a one-mm. diameter 201-thallium line source in an
average-man Rando phantom made by Alderson Research Laboratories, Inc.
The imaging system employed consisted of an Ohio-Nuclear Anger Camera
(Sigma 400) interfaced to a DEC PDP-11 computer using a DEC Gamma-11
interface. The measured 99mTc performance parameters for the system
were 3.8 mm. FWHM intrinsic spatial resolution and 12% FWHM energy
resolution. Measurements of the 201-thallium line spread function were
determined for the Ohio-Nuclear high-resolution collimator and the medium-
sensitivity collimator in the anterior, LAO 45°, and lateral projections.
A 20% photopeak window centered around the predominant x-ray emissions of
201-thallium was employed with data collected in one-mm. pixels.
The results of these measurements are summarized in Table 1 and Figure 3.
The results compare favorably with previous measurements of
201-thallium resolution (1,2,23). In particular, the 8.9 mm. FWHM
obtained with the high-resolution collimator when compared with the 18.7 mm.
value obtained by Atkins (1) demonstrates the marked improvement in imaging
performance that has occurred in recent years (2). It is notable that the
medium-sensitivity collimator increases the FWHM by only 1.4 mm. in the
anterior and LAO views while providing improvements in sensitivity of
greater than a factor of two.

The spread function measured with the medium-sensitivity collimator
in the anterior projection was used to define the smoothing filter. The
line spread function was first forced to a shape symmetric about its
first moment so that the Fourier transformation would have no imaginary
components. The real coefficients were then set to zero for all frequencies
above the first zero crossing. All coefficients so adjusted had
normalized values of less than .005. The shape of the filter is

illustrated in Figure 4 for values of n = 1, 3, 6, 10, 20, and 50.
The images from two case studies with four views each were processed
using filters corresponding to these six values of n. On the basis of
these images a value of n = 3 was selected. For comparison purposes, the
smoothing filter is plotted in Figure 5 along with the noise spectrum
corresponding to an information density of 800 counts/cm.^{2} recorded
in 4-mm. pixels, and the signal spectrum of a Gaussian-shaped lesion
20-mm. in diameter. It should be noted that the maximum observable
frequency afforded by sampling with 4-mm. pixels (i.e. a 64 X 64 matrix

TABLE I

Measured 201-thallium Resolution and Sensitivity

	High-Resolution Collimator*		Medium-Sensitivity Collimator*	
	FWHM,MM**	SENSITIVITY***	FWHM,MM**	SENSITIVITY***
Anterior	8.9	1.00	10.3	2.50
LAO 45	8.9	1.08	10.3	2.68
Lateral	10.7	.79	13.8	1.95

     * Ohio-Nuclear, Inc.
    ** Full Width at Half Maximum of the measured line spread
       function (see text).
   *** Sensitivity relative to the high-resolution collimator in
       the anterior view.

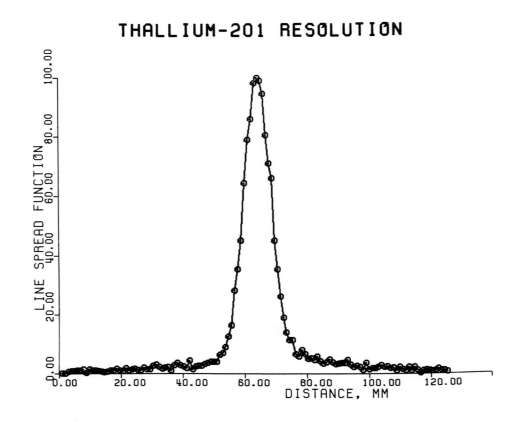

FIG. 3. Thallium-201 line spread function measured with a medium sensitivity collimator in the anterior projection using an average man RANDO phantom.

with a 10" field of view) is .125 cycles/mm. (6,17) which is slightly
above the zero point in the thallium transfer function.

   The effect of the image smoothing algorithm is illustrated in
Figure 6 where image data which has been operated on by the spatially
variant background subtraction algorithm is shown before and after smoothing.
The smoothing algorithm does not cause oscillation such as produced by
a sharp frequency cutoff and does not degrade the image resolution as
does the commonly employed nine-point weighted smoothing algorithm.
The algorithm is programmed in Fortran and, using a published version of
the fast Fourier transform (17), requires approximately 4 minutes per
view on the authors' computer. Our initial experience with the algorithm
suggests that it is effective in minimizing the influence of statistical
noise on observer response.

MOTION CORRECTION

   Optimized spatial detail in static myocardial images requires that
the degrading effects of myocardial motion be minimized. The extent of
motion in 201-thallium myocardial images may be appreciated by observing
a multi-gated 201-thallium examination with instrumentation as employed
for left ventricular blood pool studies(24,25). Improved static images
may be obtained by rejecting image data during those time intervals when
the ventricular wall is in motion.

   The motion of the myocardial wall during the cardiac cycle is
complex. Estimates of ventricular volume are well performed by nuclear
medicine blood pool studies or cardiac angiography, but the wall motions
observed are exaggerated since the wall thickness increases by about
5 mm. during contraction and movement of chamber fluid in the axial
direction is by a squeezing action (26). Another estimate of wall
motion may be made by measuring the movement of coronary arteries
with coronary angiograms. Observations in our department on the motion of
the left circumflex artery and the left anterior descending artery
suggest a motion amplitude of 10 mm. A more precise description of
the time motion profile of the ventricular wall can be made by observing
the position of the posterior ventricular wall on an M-mode echo-
cardiograph (Figure 7). The ventricular wall remains relatively
stationary during approximately one-half of the cardiac cycle and rapidly
contracts and relaxes during the remaining half. For the case
illustrated the amplitude of wall motion is 7 mm. at the outer wall
and 12 mm. at the inner wall with the average motion amplitude equal to
9 mm. The wall motion will, of course, depend on a variety of physiologic
parameters reflecting heart motion including heart rate, chamber volume,
and ejection fraction.

   The image blurring produced by the average myocardial motion illustrated in Figure 7 can be analyzed by determining the distribution
function of myocardial positions (i.e., determining the length of time
for which the myocardial position remains within a small interval). This
function, illustrated in Figure 7, may be interpreted as the resolution
spread function for motion degradation. The convolution of this function
with the system line spread function (Figure 3) yields the effective
line spread function including contributions from motion. An approximate

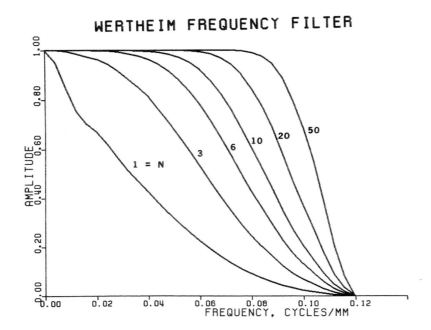

FIG. 4. The Wertheim frequency filter is illustrated as a function of n. For n equals 1, the filter is equal to the modulation transfer function computed from the line spread function illustrated in Fig. 3.

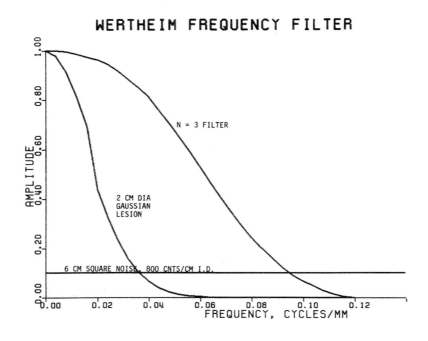

FIG. 5. The frequency filter used for smoothing thallium-201 myocardial images is illustrated (n = 3) along with the spectrum of a 2-cm-diameter Gaussian lesion and the noise spectrum.

calculation indicates that the width of the spread function is increased
by 5 to 6 mm. due to the effects of myocardial wall motion for the case
illustrated in Figure 7.

To remove the image motion degradation, we have suppressed image
data collection during a specific time interval. A window equal to 50%
of the R-R interval is centered about a point just after the T wave. The
gate interval and its effect on the motion
spread function is noted in Figure 7.   Image blurring with the synchronized data suppression is reduced to less than 1 mm. The gating procedure
may be accomplished by selectively adding the appropriate frames of a
multi-gated patient study or by collecting a static frame using a
modified cardiac synchronizer. The loss of 50% of the image data due to
motion correction is compensated by our use of a medium-sensitivity
collimator and thus the total imaging time is equivalent to that of a
conventional examination performed with a high-resolution collimator.
The improvement of 5-6 mm. in resolution accomplished by motion correction
more than offsets the 1-mm. loss of resolution introduced by using the medium-
sensitivity   collimator   rather than the high-resolution collimator.

The results of this motion correction are illustrated in Figure 8
where the LAO 40⁰ view of a patient study is shown with and without motion
correction. Data for these two images were collected simultaneously with
the uncorrected view having a maximum information density of 1600
counts/sq. cm. and the motion-corrected image having a maximum information
density of 800 counts/sq. cm. Both images have been processed with the
spatially variant background and Wertheim filtering algorithms. In
general, the motion corrected images demonstrate a larger heart size,
thinner wall dimensions, and decreased signal level in the center portion of
the image when compared with uncorrected studies. We have to date evaluated
only a limited number of cases using motion correction. Our preliminary
experience suggests that motion correction is an important element in
optimizing 201-thallium image quality.

RESULTS

The image processing techniques described are now being performed
routinely for all 201-thallium examinations in our department. For stress
examinations imaging is begun 5 minutes following an intravenous injection;
the average time per view is 8 minutes. Images are collected for a maximum
cardiac I.D. of 1600 counts/sq. cm. leaving a maximum of 800 counts/sq. cm.
for the motion-corrected images. Anterior, LAO 40⁰, LAO 60⁰, and lateral
views are routinely obtained. Image processing,which requires approximately
50 minutes per case,is done overnight by using the DEC RT-11 batch program.
Processed and unprocessed computer generated images displayed on a black
and white monitor are recorded on KODAK SO 179 film.

The effectiveness of background subtraction and smoothing was analyzed
by studying 21 cases for which stress EKG and coronary angiograms were
available. Processed and unprocessed images were read by three observers
of varying experience. While enough statistical information has not been
obtained to make a definitive statement, it appears that there is an
improvement in the trained observer's response to the processed images.
Our experience with motion corrected images is also limited. Illustrated

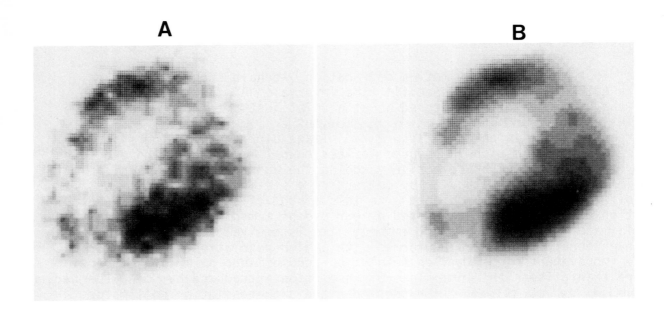

FIG. 6. The effect of the image smoothing algorithm described is illustrated before (A) and after (B) smoothing with image data which has been operated on by the spatially variant background subtraction algorithm (the same data as shown in Fig. 2).

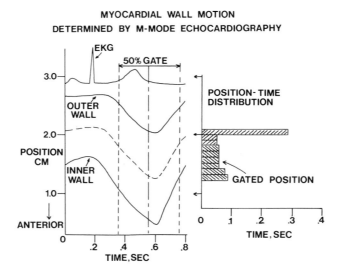

FIG. 7. The time motion profile of the ventricular wall as determined from an M-mode echocardiogram is shown at left. The distribution function of myocardial position is illustrated at right.

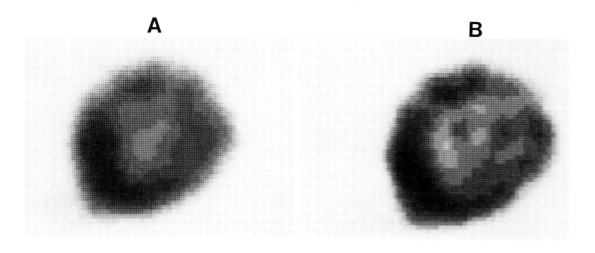

FIG. 8. The LAO 40° view of a patient study is shown with (A) and without (B) motion correction. The uncorrected image has an information density of 1600 cts/cm^2 and the motion corrected image has an information density of 800 cts/cm^2.

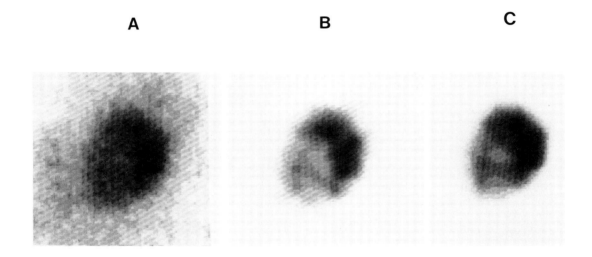

FIG. 9. Image data after background subtraction, smoothing, and motion correction for a case with abnormal stress findings shown in LAO 40° projection. The same data is shown in (C) without motion correction.

in Figure 9 is a case with abnormal stress findings for which the LAO 40°
view is shown. Demonstration of the underperfused area apprears improved
on the computer processed image when compared to the original data.
The final determination of whether improved lesion detectability results
from the image processing techniques described here will require more
extensive observer response studies

REFERENCES

1. Atkins, H.L., et al: "Thallium-201 for Medical Use. Part 3: Human
    Distribution and Physical Imaging Properties", J. Nucl. Med., 18: 133-
    140, 1977.

2. Hoogland, D., et al: "Thallium-201 Imaging Capabilities of Scintillation
    Cameras in Community Hospitals", J. Nucl. Med., 18: 640, 1977.

3. Goris, Michael L., et al: "Interpolative Background Subtraction",
    J. Nucl. Med. 17: 744-747, 1976.

4. Narahara, Kenneth A., et al: "Myocardial Imaging with Thallium-201: An
    Experimental Model for Analysis of the True Myocardial and Background
    Image Components", J. Nucl. Med. 18: 781-786, 1977.

5. DeGraff, C.N., et al: "A Refocussing Filter Based on Fridman's Theorem,
    Applied to Tl-201 Myocardial Scintigrams, in Proceedings of the IVth
    Intern. Conf. on Information Processing in Scintigraphy, Orsay, July,
    1975.

6. Brown, D.W. et al: "Quantification of the Radionuclide Scan", Seminars
    in Nuclear Medicine, Vol. 3, No. 4, 1973.

7. Brown, D.W.: "Computer Processing of Scans Using Fourier and Other
    Transformations", J. Nucl. Med., Vol. 12, No. 6, 287-291, 1971.

8. Buzzi, K.W.: "Digital Low-Pass Filtering", J. Nucl. Med., 17: 844-
    846, 1976.

9. Sebern, M.J., et al: "Minicomputer Enhancement of Scintillation
    Camera Images Using Fast Fourier Transform Techniques", J. Nucl. Med.
    17: 647-652, 1976.

10. Metz, C.E. and Beck, R.N.: "Quantitative Effects of Stationary Linear
    Image Processing on Noise and Resolution of Structure in Radionuclide
    Images", J. Nucl. Med., Vol. 15, No. 3, 164-170, 1974.

11. Gustafsson, T.R. and Pizer, S.M., "Non-Stationary Metz-Filtering",
    in Proceedings of the IVth Intern. Conf. on Information Processing
    in Scintigraphy, Orsay, July, 1975.

12. Gallagher, Joe H., and Preston, D.F.: "The Annihilation Transform - A New Image Smoothing Technique", Proceedings of Seventh Symposium on Sharing of Computer Programs and Technology in Nuclear Medicine, Computer Assisted Data Processing, CONF - 770101, ERDA, 1977.

13. Bell, P.R. et al: "Non-Linear Image Processing", in Proceedings of the Sixth Symposium on Sharing of Computer Programs and Technology in Nuclear Medicine, Society of Nuclear Medicine, 1976.

14. Kirch, D.L.: "Nonlinear Digital Techniques for Enhancement of Radionuclide Images", J. Nucl. Med. 13: 311-325, 1973.

15. Inovye, T. et al: "Computer Method for Processing Scintillation Camera Images", J. Nucl. Med., Vol. 14: No. 6, 1973.

16. Harmon, L.D. and Julesz, B.: "Masking in Visual Recognition: Effects of Two-Dimensional Filtered Noise", Science, Vol. 180, 1194-1197, 1973.

17. Brigham, E. Oran: The Fast Fourier Transform, Prentice-Hall, Inc., 1974.

18. Pizer, S.M. and Todd-Pokropek, A.E., "Noise Character in Processed Scintigrams", in Proceedings of the IVth Intern. Conf. on Information Processing in Scintigraphy, Orsay, July, 1975.

19. Wertheim, G.K., "Novel Smoothing Algorithm", Rev. Sci. Instrum., Vol. 46, No. 10, Oct. 1975.

20. Marchand, E.W.: "Derivation of the Point Spread Function from the Line Spread Function", J. of the Optical Society of America, Vol. 54, No. 7, 915-919, 1964.

21. Marchand, E.W.: "From Line to Point Spread Function: The General Case", J. of the Optical Society of America, Vol. 55, No. 4, 352-354, 1965.

22. Swindell, W. and Barrett, H.: "Computerized Tomography: Taking Sectional X-rays", Physics Today, Vol. 30, No. 12, 1977, Pg. 35.

23. Graham, S.L.: "Collimation for Imaging the Myocardium II", J. Nucl. Med. 17: 719-723, 1976.

24. Wagner, H.N. et al: "Computer-Assisted Cinematic Displays in Nuclear Medicine", J. Nucl. Med. 18: 615, 1977.

25. Cascade, P.N.: "Thallium-201 Myocardial Studies with Multiple ECG Gated Images and Movie Display", Circulation, Vols: 55 and 56, Supp. III, Oct. 1977.

26. Mirsky, Ghista, and Sandler: "Cardiac Mechanics: Physiological, Clinical and Mathematical Consideration, John Wiley and Sons.

A FIRST PASS RADIONUCLIDE METHOD FOR ESTIMATING EJECTION FRACTION AT REST AND DURING EXERCISE

Jyrki T. Kuikka

Division of Nuclear Medicine
Department of Clinical Chemistry
University Central Hospital
SF-90220 Oulu 22, Finland

ABSTRACT

A low-frequency radionuclide technique is described for evaluating the ejection fraction both at rest and during muscular exercise. Technetium-99m as human serum albumin is intravenously injected and the heart is imaged in the 30° LAO position with a scintillation camera interfaced to a digital computer and a read-out system. Time-activity curves extracted from the regions of the heart and lungs are analyzed by fitting sets of gamma-variate functions to the observed curves. Thirty-two healthy volunteers were studied and the analyses yielded the following values for the left ventricular ejection fraction: 67 ± 8 % (mean ± S.D.) at rest, 74 ± 8 % during mild exercise, 79 ± 5 % during moderate exercise and 80 ± 4 % during heavy exercise. Uneven mixing of the tracer with ventricular blood and the effects of background correction are also discussed. The method presented gives results with a reproducibility of 16 % (mean of the differences ± 2xS.D.) and an accuracy of 29 %.

INTRODUCTION

Changes in left ventricular dynamics caused by muscular exercise are usual in daily life. Examination of these changes, however, requires that methods are not harmful to the exercising subjects during the investigation. Several radionuclide methods (1-7) have been published, but only rarely are these methods usable for exercise measurements (1,6,7).

The evaluation of left ventricular function during exercise by using tracer dilution techniques is complicated by: (1) movement of the exercising subject, (2) "cross-talk detection" caused by external measurement, (3) frame-time limitation, (4) statistical counting noise, (5) tracer dispersion, (6) recirculation, (7) lack of homogenous mixing of tracer within the chamber, and (8) count-volume non-linearity.

In the present study the suitability of low-frequency radiocardiography, RCG, (frame time = 0.2-0.5 sec) has been investigated both at rest and during leg exercise. The results obtained from 32 healthy volunteers are also presented.

DATA ACQUISITION PROTOCOL

A small bolus containing 3-10 mCi of technetium-99m as human serum albumin (or indium-113m as transferrin) is rapidly injected into an antecubital vein and immediately flushed with 10 ml of saline. The bolus flow through the heart and lungs is imaged with a scintillation camera (RADICAMERA II) interfaced to a small digital computer (NOVA 1220, 24k of core) and a read-out system (NUKAB) using a fast television technique. The camera head with a high-resolution parallel-hole collimator is oriented in the left anterior oblique position (30° LAO). The frame time used is 0.2-0.5 sec depending on the heart rate of the subject {i.e. $\Delta t \simeq 60$ sec/(2xheart rate)}. The 128 images digitized on a 128x128 matrix are gathered and corrected for uniformity, and then stored on a magnetic disc for subsequent computer analysis. Data correction and transferral takes about 1.5 minutes of computer time. The following regions of interest (ROI) are selected using a light-pen: (1) superior vena cava (in order to confirm the arrival of a sharp and compact bolus to the heart), (2) right ventricle, (3) left ventricle, and (4) whole heart. Nine regions can be selected at the same time if needed. The time-activity curves are displayed on a color TV-monitor, printed out and transferred into a central purpose computer (NOVA 840, 64k of core) for processing.

DATA HANDLING

The objective of the data manipulations is to fit a unimodal density function of specific form to the time-activity curve obtained during dilution process. Thompson et al (8) have previously fitted tracer dilution curves obtained after intravenous injection with a gamma-variate function, a smooth, right-skewed function:

$$C(t) = K \cdot (t - T)^a \cdot e^{-(t - T)/b} \tag{1}$$

where K is the scale constant (K = 0, when $t \leq T$), T the appearance time, and a and b are gamma fitting parameters. The appearance time is defined as that time after the injection of the tracer when the measured tracer concentration exceeds the mean plus four standard deviations of the background concentration. The terminating point of the fitting procedure on the downslope of the dilution curve is approximately equal to 70 % of the peak concentration. The data between the appearance time and the 70 % point are used in the fitting. The weighted least squares method $\{w_i = C^2(t_i)\}$ of Starmer and Clark (9) is used (Fig. 1).

FORMULATION OF MODEL

After an intravenous injection of tracer, the tracer bolus flows with widening distribution through the heart and lungs. In every part of the cardiopulmonary system the distribution of the tracer changes in a way characteristic of the location in question. Assume that the cardiopulmonary system consists of mathematically linear components in series, which are perfused by a steady flow. Then the output, $C_o(t)$, is a convolution of the input, $C_i(t)$, and the transfer function, h(t)

$$C_o(t) = C_i(t) * h(t) \tag{2}$$

where the asterisk denotes the process of convolution (10). If the input and output functions are known, the transfer function can be obtained by using a numerical deconvolution technique. The shapes of the input and output functions are assumed to be gamma-variate functions (Eq. 1). The transfer function appropriate to each pair of input/output curves is determined in terms of (1) a single exponential function and in terms of (2) a gamma-variate function. Figure 2 shows a flow diagram of data analysis.

METHODOLOGICAL DIFFICULTIES

The single exponential approximation assumes that the cardiac chamber is a pure mixing chamber and the gamma-variate approximation is a combination of mixing chamber and delay line. Figure 3 shows that the single exponential model gives an accurate fit to the descending part of the output curve, but fails greatly in the fitting of the ascending part of the curve. This finding suggests that the tracer is not uniformly mixed with the blood in the ventricle.

Fourteen right atrial/ventricular time-activity curves were analyzed in order to look for a possible difference between the volume values calculated from the single exponential function

$$RV(exp) = FSV / FEF = FSV / (1 - e^{-kt}) \tag{3A}$$

and from the gamma-variate function

$$RV(gam) = SF \cdot \bar{t} + \frac{1}{2} \cdot FSV \tag{3B}$$

where FSV is the forward stroke volume (i.e. systemic flow, SF, divided by the heart rate, HR), FEF the forward ejection fraction, k the transfer rate constant describing the mean emptying rate of the activity from the ventricle, and $\bar{t}$ is the transit time

$$\bar{t} = MTT(out) - MTT(in) \tag{3C}$$

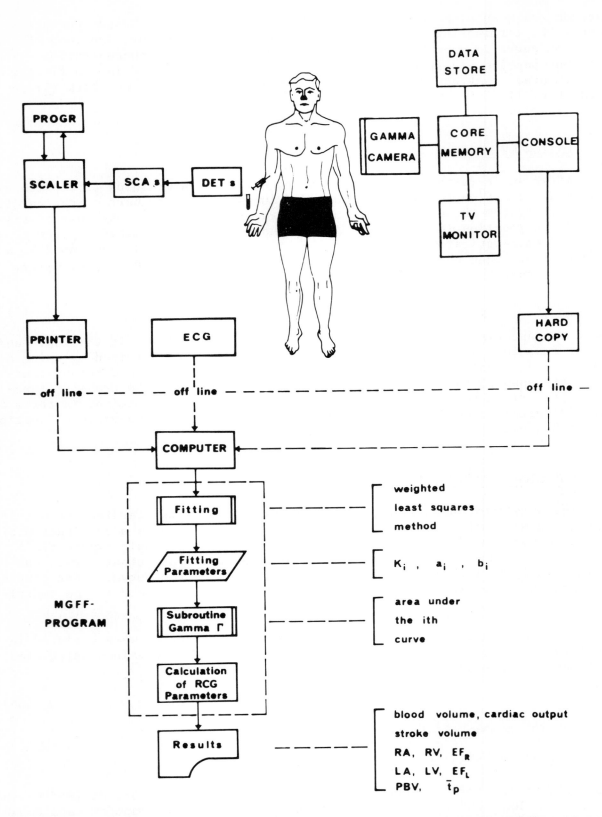

FIG. 1. Flow chart of the measurement system, and data manipulation by computer. MGFF = modified gamma function fitting. This picture is similar to a picture published in Nuclear Medicine (Ref. 7).

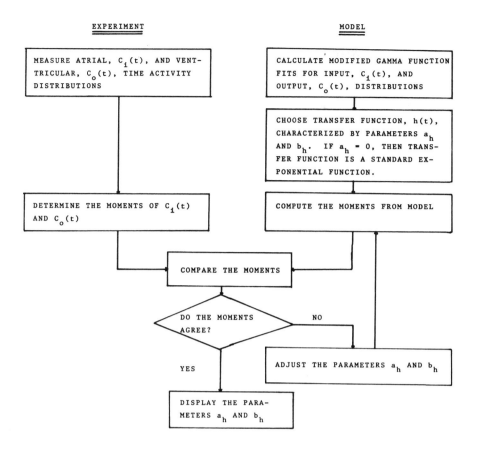

FIG. 2. A flow diagram of data analysis of measured atrial and ventricular time-activity distributions in terms of model expressed by functions $C_i(t)$ and $C_o(t) = C_i(t)*h(t)$. The convolution integral is calculated by using Simpson's approximation method with a step of $\Delta t/4$.

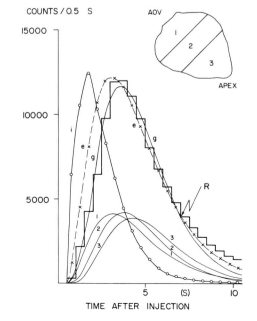

FIG. 3. Use of a single exponential function (e) and a gamma function (g) as the transfer function for the left ventricle. The curves 1, 2, and 3 show the variation of the activity distributions in the ventricle. Note a poor mixing and time delay in the apex area. i = input curve.

A comparison yielded a regression equation of

$$RV(exp) = 0.89 \cdot RV(gam) - 11 \text{ ml} \quad ; \quad r = 0.88$$

and

$$RV(exp) / RV(gam) = 0.84 \pm 0.13 \quad ; \quad p < 0.001 \quad \text{(paired t-test)}$$

An additional study was also undertaken. The whole area of the ventricle (Fig. 3) was divided into 3 parts and the curves were analyzed using the gamma-variate function as a model. The transit times and relative dispersions (i.e. standard deviation of the density function of transit times divided by the mean transit time) show clearly uneven mixing of tracer in the ventricle, with the minimum mixing in the apex area and the maximum mixing near the aortic valve, while the transit time in the apex area is also much longer (40 %) than that in the upper part of the ventricle. The above shows that a single cardiac chamber is not well described by a pure mixing chamber model.

The counts detected externally from the region of interest are composed of the counts from this chamber, the counts from the overlapping regions, as well as from scattered radiation from the adjacent regions. This background is low for the right ventricle, but increases significantly, when the left ventricle is studied, being on the order of 30-50 % of the total counts observed (Fig. 4). Both explicit (11,12) and empirical (13,14) approaches are used for eliminating background counts. The input/output pairs of the time activity curves are measured and a transit time between them is calculated (Eq. 3C). In the empirical approaches the background curve is generated representing background radioactivity from aorta, left atrium, lungs, right heart, recirculation, and incomplete mixing of tracer within the ventricle.

The effect of background on forward ejection fraction/end-diastolic volume was studied by the technique described by Steele et al. (13). The background curve extracted from the semiannular ring surrounding the chamber of interest is multiplied so that its tail is tangential to that of the uncorrected chamber dilution curve. The descending part of the resultant background-corrected curve is then fitted with a single exponential function. End-diastolic volume is calculated and compared to the figure obtained from the transit time principle (Eq. 3B). The single exponential analysis yielded larger end-diastolic volume values throughout the material than the transit time principle, being on the average 1.2xRV(gam) for the right ventricle and 1.21xRV(gam) for the left. The corresponding ejection fraction estimates are about 20 % less than those obtained from the transit time principle.

One critical source of error in ejection fraction/end-diastolic volume calculations is a low count rate with a large statistical deviation (S.D.) Since the detected amount of activity is dependent on the flow rate through the chamber, volume of the chamber, input distribution (and injection technique), frame time and of course on the equipment and radionuclide used, at high heart rate and flow levels the statistical counting noise increases greatly. Figure 5 shows dependence of the count rate on flow (SF = 1xF, 2xF, and 3xF) and on frame time (Δt = 0.50, 0.25, and 0.15 sec). When the frame time is about 1/3 of the frame time at rest and the flow is about 3 times the flow at rest, the count rate is diminished by nearly $(1/3)^2$, $\propto 1/9$ of the count rate at rest. This effect is not very critical in low frequency studies (Δt =

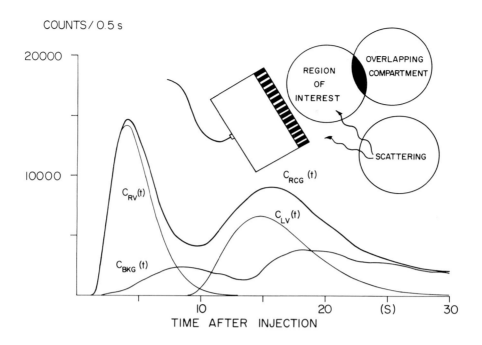

FIG. 4. Time-activity curves extracted from the regions of the right and left ventricle (RCG) and background (BKG). A single exponential fit to the descending part of the background-corrected curve (LV) yielded too low ejection fraction (22% vs. 38% as obtained from gamma function fit).

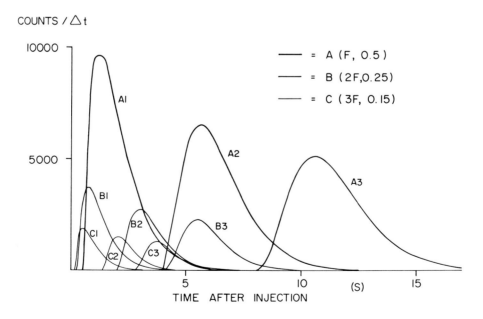

FIG. 5. Effect of flow (SF = 1xF, 2xF, and 3xF), input distribution (width of $C_i(t)$ = 1x, 2x, and 3x initial tracer distribution) and frame time (Δt = 0.50, 0.25, and 0.15 sec) to the count rate. The thick lines represent a flow of 6 l/min, the medium 12 l/min, and the thin 18 l/min.

0.2-0.5 sec), the maximum errors (assume: statistical counting noise = 4xS.D.) in volume values being 3.5 %, 4.4 % and 6.8 % in the corresponding order of the flow, 1xF, 2xF and 3xF. In the first pass, beat-by-beat, technique, the statistical counting noise is the limiting factor at high flows (SF > 7 1/min/m^2) and heart rates (HR > 130 b/min), making ejection fraction determinations less reliable than at rest.

Calculations of mean transit time (Eq. 3C) and from it, chamber volume (Eq. 3B), are not practical, because the fluctuations in volume and flow are occuring at intervals that are not greatly less than the mean transit time and create the possibility of large errors. Even if the flow were steady, the method demands high count rate and accurate determinations of the regions of interest (narrow areas both just the input and output ends of the ventricle).

We used an empirical formula for forward ejection fraction calculations based on a dispersion relation (7,15). The width of the input distribution is directly estimated through the parameters obtained from the modified gamma function fitting, MGFF, of the ventricular time activity curve. The transfer rate constant, k, in equation 3A should be rewritten as

$$FEF = 1 - e^{-kt} \simeq 1 - e^{-(0.693/T_{1/2})\cdot(60/HR)} \tag{4}$$

where

$$T_{1/2} = T_{1/2}(out) - T_{1/2}(in) \simeq b\cdot\{1 - f\cdot(a + 1)^{-1/2}\} \tag{5}$$

in which a and b are gamma fitting parameters (Eq. 1), and

$$f = 1 + e^{-\{T + b\cdot(a + 1)\}/T} \tag{6}$$

is the experimental correction factor determined from the physical flow model (15).   Equations 1, 4, 5 and 6 allow rapid and easy computation of ejection fraction from the measured ventricular time activity curve. The method is relatively independent of the starting (T) and terminating (TT) points. If these points are incorrectly located (i.e. T = T ± Δt, and/or TT = TT ± Δt), the inaccuracy of FEF will be on the order of 5 %.

CLINICAL STUDIES

The test subjects were 32 healthy volunteers. The mean age was 27 years (range 19 to 47 years). The measurements were made in supine position on a special table equipped with shoulder pads. 76 runs were carried out, 32 at rest and 44 during leg exercise.

The changes in the means and standard deviations of cardiac index, left ventricular ejection fraction and pulmonary capillary pressure at rest, during mild exercise, during moderate exercise and during heavy exercise are seen in Fig. 6. Pulmonary capillary pressure is calculated from the two-peaked radio-cardiogram using the multi-linear regression equation previously described by di Matteo et al. (16). Pulmonary capillary pressure, forward ejection fraction and forward stroke volume seem to be the most promising indices for e-valuation of cardiac function from the radiocardiograms (Kuikka et al.: unpublished data).

The reproducibility of the method (end-diastolic volume) was tested in 19 healthy subjects by making duplicate measurements at an interval of 15 minutes. The correlation coefficient was 0.96 and the mean of the differences was 1 % with a standard deviation of 7 % (Fig. 7A).

The accuracy of the method was studied in 15 cardiac patients who also underwent left ventricular cineangiocardiography. A comparison of radionuclide and cineangiographic left ventricular end-diastolic volumes yielded a correlation coefficient of 0.95 using a quadratic regression equation (Fig. 7B). The quadratic regression equation is probably due to self attenuation of radionuclide or some discrepancy between the ellipsoid model and the true ventricular shape, since the contour of the ventricle is both irregular and alternating. The mean of the differences was 3 % with a standard deviation of 13 %. On the basis of the determinations it can be calculated that the 95 % significance limit of the reproducibility is ± 16 % for the end-diastolic volume. The corresponding accuracy limit is ± 29 %.

CONCLUSION

Low frequency ($\Delta t = 0.2$–0.5 sec) counting is sufficiently accurate to permit a weighted least squares fit using 15-20 data points. Inaccuracy in the calculation of the transfer rate constant (ejection fraction) introduced from statistical counting noise is certainly less than ± 10 % with a peak count rate of 1000 counts/channel.

A specific function of time is used for fitting time activity curves and forward ejection fraction/end-diastolic volume is directly derived from a simple mathematical relation. However, it should be emphasize that the volume values calculated are not exactly anatomical volumes, but rather functional volumes or so called volume indices. An error as great as 20 to 30 % may occur. This is understandable considering the assumptions on which the equations are based. These include linearity, steady flow, instantaneous mixing and time invariance; moreover the recirculation and input distribution approximations employed are empirical.

The methods used in hospitals are always specific to a given hospital, because methods of analyses are not standardized. For example the mean values of normal left ventricular ejection fraction vary at rest from 50 to 70 % (see also Fig. 6) depending on the methods and equipment used. However, the noninvasive radionuclide methods give extremely valuable information in patient management and care. The techniques are relatively simple and can be performed repeatedly both at rest and during exercise.

ACKNOWLEDGEMENTS

The author is grateful to Dr. J. Timisjärvi for his valuable collaboration in a part of this work. Drs. J.B. Bassingthwaighte and G.A. Holloway Jr contributed helpful criticisms of the content and the presentation of this work. Ms. Hedi Nurk prepared the illustrations. This investigation was supported in part by a Public Health Service International Research Fellowship (F05 TW0248 01-01).

The present address: Center for Bioengineering, RF-52, University of Washington, Seattle, WA98195, U.S.A.

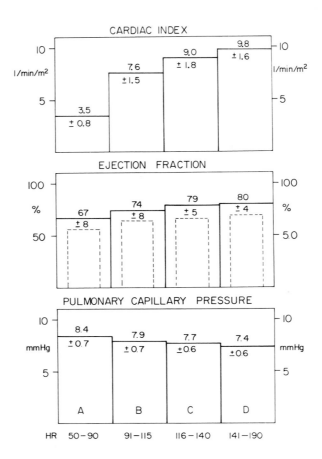

FIG. 6. Mean values and standard deviations obtained from 32 healthy subjects at rest (A) and during exercises (B, C, and D). The mean heart rates are 66 + 10, 103 + 8, 129 + 7, and 155 + 10 b/min. The dashed lines show the mean ejection fraction estimated from the study of Borer et al.

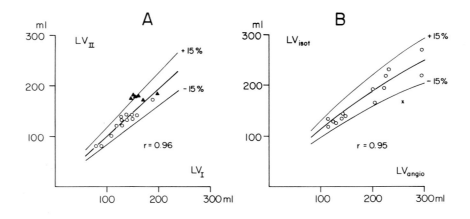

FIG. 7. (A) Reproducibility of the radiocardiography. ○ = at rest and ▲ = during exercise. (B) Comparison of left ventricular and end-diastolic volumes between radiocardiography and cineangiography. x = fibrillating heart rate (excluded from the fitting of regression curve).

REFERENCES

1. de VERNEJOUL P, DELALOYE B, di GREGORIO V, et al.: Mesure du débit cardiaque et des volumes ventriculaires par radiocardiographie. Rev. Franç. Etud. Clin. Biol. 9: 693-715, 1964

2. HEISKANEN T: Analogue model for the analysis of radiocardiograms. Cardiovascular Res. 5: 268-276, 1971

3. VAN DYKE D, ANGER HO, SULLIVAN RW, et al.: Cardiac evaluation from radioisotope dynamics. J. Nucl. Med. 13: 585-592, 1972

4. PARKER JA, SECKER-WALKER R, HILL R, et al.: A new technique for the calculation of left ventricular ejection fraction. J. Nucl. Med. 13: 649-651, 1972

5. WEBER PM, dosREMEDIOS LV, JASKO IA: Quantitative radioisotope angiocardiography. J. Nucl. Med. 13: 815-822, 1972

6. BORER JS, BACHARACH SL, GREEN MV, et al.: Real-time radionuclide cineangiography in the noninvasive evaluation of global and regional left ventricular function at rest and during exercise in patients with coronary-artery disease. N. Engl. J. Med. 296: 839-844, 1977

7. KUIKKA J: Cardiopulmonary response to muscular exercise in healthy young human subjects. Nucl. Med. 16: 137-139, 1977

8. THOMPSON HK, STARMER CF, WHALEN RE, et al.: Indicator transit time considered as gamma variate. Circ. Res. 14: 502-515, 1964

9. STARMER CF, CLARK D: Computer computations of cardiac output using the gamma function. J. Appl. Physiol. 28: 219-220, 1970

10. BASSINGTHWAIGHTE JB: Blood flow and diffusion through mammalian organs. Science 167: 1347-1353, 1970

11. ISHII Y, MACINTYRE WJ: Analytical approach to dynamic radioisotope recording. J. Nucl. Med. 12: 792-799, 1971

12. JONES RH, SABISTON DC, BATES BB, et al.: Quantitative radionuclide angiocardiography for determination of chamber to chamber cardiac transit times. Am. J. Cardiol. 30: 855-864, 1972

13. STEELE P, KIRCH DL, MATTHEWS M, et al. Measurement of left heart ejection fraction and end-diastolic volume by a computerized, scintigraphic technique using a wedged pulmonary arterial catheterer. Am. J. Cardiol. 34: 179-186, 1974

14. FOLLAND ED, HAMILTON GW, LARSON SM, et al.: The radionuclide ejection fraction: A comparison of three radionuclide techniques with contrast angiography. J. Nucl. Med. 18: 1159-1166, 1977

15. KUIKKA J: $^{113}In^m$ radiocardiographic measurements of cardiopulmonary parameters in healthy subjects and in cardiac patients. (Ph.D. thesis) Department of Physics, University of Jyväskylä, Jyväskylä, Finland, Res. Rep. No. 2/1976

16. di MATTEO J, VACHERON A, MEILHAC B, et al.: Mesure des pressions pulmonaires moyennes et de la pression ventriculaire droite systolique par radiocardiographie. Arch. Mal. Coeur. 68: 3-9, 1975

DECONTAMINATION OF REGION OF INTEREST CURVES
USING MODELS OF THE CENTRAL CIRCULATION

Jordan L. Spencer

Alba Regina

Frank S. Castellana

Department of Chemical Engineering and
Applied Chemistry, School of Engineering
and Applied Science, Columbia University
New York, New York   10027

Marvin I. Friedman

and

Richard N. Pierson, Jr.

St. Luke's Hospital Center
Columbia University
New York, New York   10025

ABSTRACT

Mathematical models of the central circulation have been used to analyze ROI time-activity curves from radiocardiography studies. Both continuous flow models (constant volume chambers) and pulsatile flow (variable volume chamber) models have been employed. These models contain as undetermined parameters chamber volumes, and also crosstalk coefficients which account for the contribution to the count rate in one region-of-interest (ROI) from tracer located in chambers assigned to other regions-of-interest. The parameters of the models are determined by using iterative nonlinear regression programs which produce a weighted simultaneous least-squares fit to ROI curves corresponding to several chambers. Based on the values of the crosstalk coefficients so determined, ROI curves free of crosstalk can be estimated. Initial results are promising, although the possibility of having nonunique solutions in certain cases has to be investigated carefully.

INTRODUCTION

Region-of-interest (ROI) time-activity curves obtained in gamma camera radio-cardiography contain information on many parameters of the central circulation, parameters such as the diastolic and systolic volumes of each chamber, and flows related to shunts and valvular insufficiency if these are present. The anatomy of the heart and lungs and the nature of the available counting systems make it impossible to obtain ROI curves in which the count rate in a given ROI depends only on the amount of tracer in the chamber assigned to that ROI. Thus any method of analysis, and particularly methods designed to extract large amounts of information from the data, must take into account the background, crosstalk, or contamination which is inherent in the ROI curves to be analyzed.

In what follows we will discuss a method of analysis based on the use of mathematical models of the central circulation. These models contain as undetermined parameters not only chamber volumes, but also crosstalk coefficients which relate the count rate in a given ROI to the activity in each chamber of the heart (and lung). The parameters are determined by nonlinear regression programs which provide a weighted least-squares fit to one or more ROI curves. The crosstalk coefficients so determined can be used to calculate estimates of the ROI curves as they would appear in the absence of crosstalk, thus effecting a "decontamination" of the ROI curves.

MODELS AND PARAMETER DETERMINATION

A specific model is defined, first, by the chambers or regions of the heart or lungs which are used to represent the transient movement of tracer through the central circulation and second, by the number of ROIs and the selection of crosstalk coefficients.

If all chamber volumes and the blood flow rate are assumed constant, we call the model a continuous flow model. If certain chamber volumes and the blood flow rate vary periodically, we call the model a pulsatile flow model. Figure 1 shows a continuous flow model and a pulsatile flow model. In these models all chambers are assumed well mixed. In the pulsatile flow model the right ventricle (RV) and the left ventricle (LV) volumes vary linearly with time, filling in 70% and emptying in 30% of the cardiac cycle. The blood discharged during systole by the right ventricle is absorbed by the variable volume lung pool whose volume also varies linearly with time. The undetermined chamber volumes are denoted by B_1, B_2, ..., and the crosstalk coefficients are denoted by C_{11}, C_{12}, ... Z_1 and Z_2 are RV and LV ROI time-activity data. In the continuous flow models the cardiac output is assumed known, and in the pulsatile flow models the stroke volume and frequency are assumed known, their product equaling the cardiac output.

The models shown in Figure 1 are relatively simple. Figure 2 shows a more complex continuous flow model with six pools and with 12 or 13 free parameters depending on whether the lung volume is fixed or free.

The parameters of a model are determined by a general nonlinear regression program. In this program the equations which describe the evolution of the system in time are assumed to be of the form

$$\frac{dx}{dt} = f(x,b) \quad , \quad x(0) = h(b)$$

where t is time, x is a vector of state variables (activities in each pool) b is a vector of parameters (pool volumes and ejection fractions) and f and g are given functions. The measured variables are assumed to be related to the state variables by an equation of the form

$$z = g(x, c)$$

where z is a vector of measured variables (ROI count rates), c is a vector of parameters, (crosstalk coefficients) and g is a given function. In a specialized version of the program f and g are linear functions, i.e.

$$f = B(b)x$$

and

$$g = C(c)x$$

where B and C are matrix functions of b and c respectively.

The parameters are adjusted iteratively so as to minimize a weighted least-squares objective function of the form

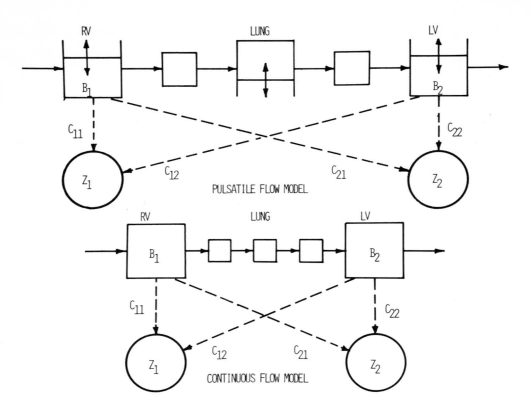

FIG. 1. Continuous flow and pulsatile flow models. (See text for notation.)

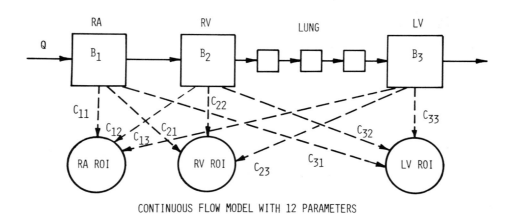

FIG. 2. Continuous flow model with 12 parameters. (See text for notation.)

$$S = \sum_{j=1}^{M} \sum_{k=1}^{N} \left\{ w_{jk} \left[z_j^*(t_k) - z_j(t_k) \right] \right\}^2$$

Here w_{jk} is the weighting coefficient for the jth measured variable z_j at the kth time t_k, and z* is a vector of measured variables. The weights are normally selected so that the data points, after weighting, have equal or approximately equal variance.

RESULTS

Initial tests of the model-based data analysis method described above were carried out using continuous flow models since continuous flow models are easily handled, and certain timing problems could arise in using pulsatile models to fit data corresponding to variable cardiac frequency. These studies were designed to test the feasibility of simultaneously determining crosstalk coefficients and chamber volumes, and to show whether models comprising a small number of well-mixed pools can adequately fit ROI time-activity curves.

In general the weights used in the nonlinear regression objective function should be selected so that the data points, after weighting, have equal variance. If the variance of the measured points is due only to counting statistics and if the errors are uncorrelated, the weights should be inversely proportional to the true value of the measured variable. As an approximation we have used weights inversely proportional to the experimental values, except that the maximum weight used was limited, to avoid excessive weights associated with very small values. Preliminary results indicate that the results are relatively insensitive to the weights.

Typical results, corresponding to the model of Figure 2, are shown in Figures 3 and 4. The data were obtained in a study involving an adult patient, and correspond to the injection of 10 millicuries of 99m-Tc HSA, using a gamma camera aligned in the RAO position. ROI time-activity data points were taken at 40-millisecond intervals, but for the initial data analysis only points 200 milliseconds apart were used. As can be seen in Figure 3 and 4, the model fits the data well, with the residuals for the RA, RV, and LV time-activity curves attributable mainly to chamber volume variations.

The parameter values determined by the nonlinear regression program are shown on a diagram of the model in Figure 5. In the model used the lung blood volume was fixed at 500 milliliters, and the cardiac output was assumed to be six liters per minute. (The pool volumes determined are proportional to the cardiac output.) The standard errors for each parameter (shown in parentheses below the parameter value) were calculated from the variance-covariance matrix and an estimate of the variance of the measurement based on the residuals. Since the residuals reflect the fact that a continuous flow model was used to fit pulsatile data, the standard errors shown may be somewhat too large. However the 95% support plane confidence limits are several times larger than the standard errors.

The chamber volumes for the right atrium, right ventricle, and left atrium were determined as 26, 104, and 169 milliliters, all of which are reasonable. As the standard errors show, the pool volumes are fairly well determined.

The crosstalk coefficients, which have meaning only as relative values, are also shown in Figure 5. The "direct" crosstalks, i.e. the RA-to-RA, RV-to-RV, and LV-to-LV coefficients, are almost equal. This is what we would expect if the ROIs are large enough to capture all (or at least the same fraction) of the counts in the respective chambers. The RV-to-LV and LV-to-RV coefficients are of the same magnitude as the direct coefficients, while the RA-to-LV and LV-to-RA coefficients are significantly smaller, again as expected for RAO data. Finally, the crosstalk coefficients have relative small standard errors, so that the possibility of simultaneously determining chamber volumes and crosstalk coefficients has been demonstrated.

Once the crosstalk coefficients are available, they can be used to generate ROI time-activity curves as they would appear if no crosstalk were present. The decontaminated curves shown in Figures 3 and 4 were obtained by setting all crosstalk coefficients except for the direct coefficients, i.e. RA-to-RA, RV-to-RA, RV-to-RV, and LV-to-LV. If the relation between the state variables x and the measured variables z is of the form

$$z = Cx$$

where C, the crosstalk matrix, is nonsingular, then

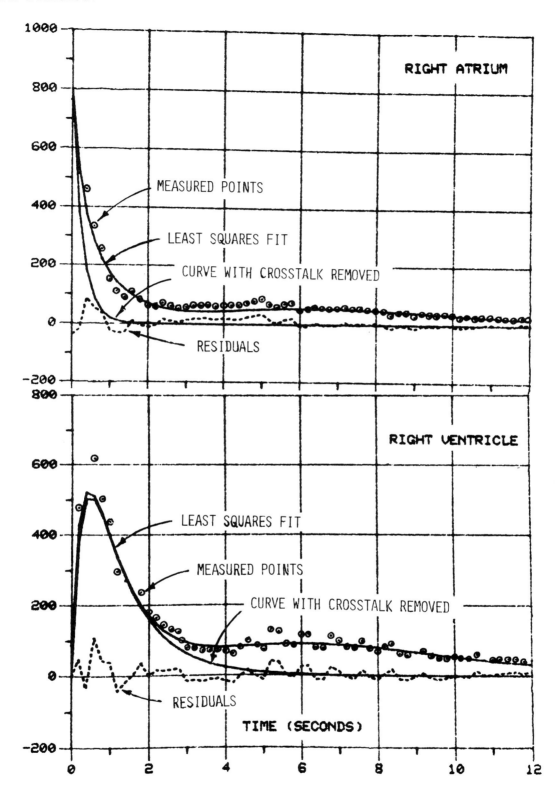

FIG. 3. Least squares fit to right atrial and right ventricular ROI time-activity curves.

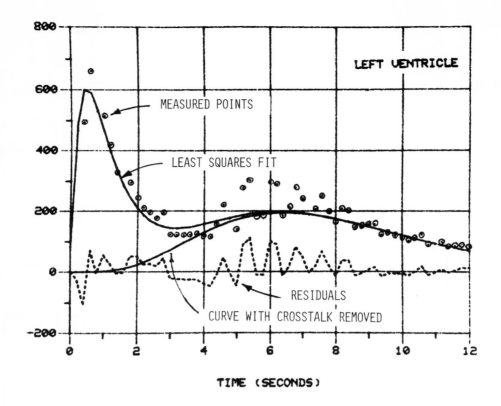

FIG. 4. Least squares fit to left ventricle ROI time-activity curves.

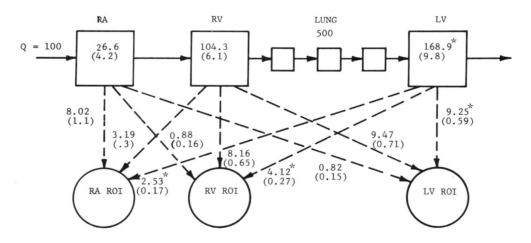

FIG. 5. Least squares parameter values and standard errors for continuous flow model.

$$x = C^{-1} z \;.$$

Thus the inverse of C can be used to generate decontaminated ROI curves from the actual ROI curves. The curves so generated will retain the effects of pulsality and counting statistics, and the decontaminated LV curve could be used, for example, to estimate ejection fraction in the usual way. Thus it is possible to use a continuous flow model to determine ejection fractions.

Since the central circulation is in fact a pulsatile system, it is reasonable to assume that it is best represented by a pulsatile model, and that continuous flow models, convenient as they are to use, might produce incorrect parameter values when used to analyze data. Although the work with pulsatile models is still in the early stages, some of the initial results are of interest. Figure 6 shows the best fit of a two-pool 6-parameter continuous flow model to data generated by the two-pool 6-parameter pulsatile model. The fit is good, and the residuals resemble those seen previously. Figure 7 shows the model used to generate the data and the best-fit parameter values. Even taking into account the parameter confidence limits, the agreement is not as good as might be expected. The tentative conclusion is that pulsatile models are to be preferred, although continuous flow models are easier to use, and may be useful for preliminary investigations.

DISCUSSION

We have shown how models can be used, in conjunction with nonlinear regression methods, to generate decontaminated ROI curves and to provide estimates of parameters such as pool volumes and ejection fractions. In the application of this method there are of course problems that require careful investigation. If the model is seriously incorrect, the results are likely to be in error. If too many parameters have to be estimated, or if parameter correlation is strong, the parameters will be poorly determined.

But the potential advantages are promising and include:

1)   The method requires minimal operator intervention and is computerizable. Of course the ROI definition is still necessary.

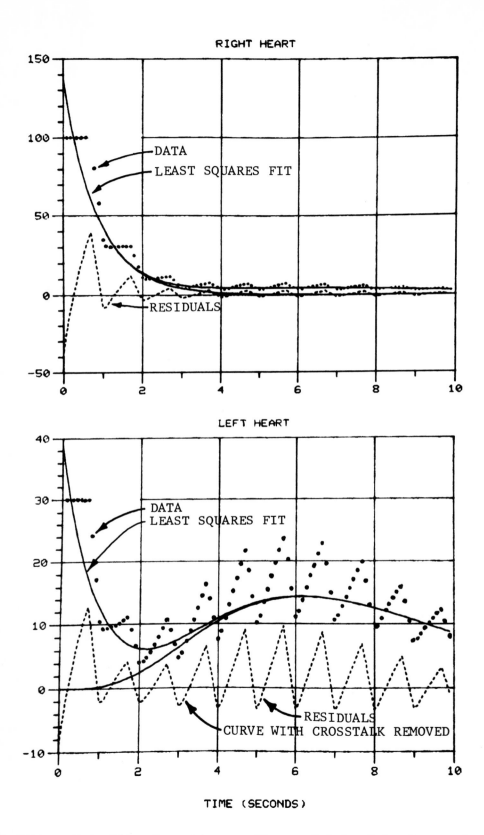

FIG. 6. Least squares fit of continuous flow model to data from pulsatile model.

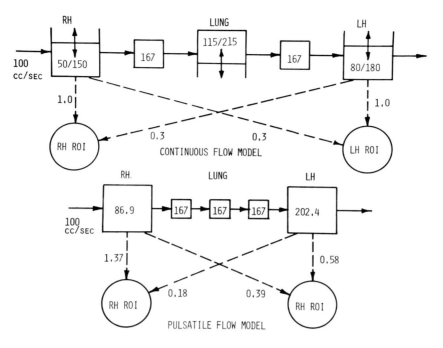

FIG. 7. Least squares parameter values for continuous flow model fit to pulsatile data.

2)   An estimate of the uncertainty in the parameter values is provided automatically. This feature may provide a method for optimizing ROI selection, in the sense that optimal ROIs should minimize the parameter confidence limits.

3)   The method provides information of interest to the physiologist and physician in addition to ejection fraction, namely volumes (or time constants) of other chambers such as right heart and lungs; detection of shunts; and evaluation of valvular insufficiency.

4)   The method provides a general and flexible framework for incorporating into the analysis procedure additional information about the system.   For example, if self-absorption varies with chamber volume in a known way, or if mixing is not complete in a chamber, these effects are easily incorporated into the model.

5)   A model based analysis of biplane data is easily developed, and takes advantage of the fact that chambers that overlap in one view may be well separated in another.

AUTOMATIC, DISPLAY INTERACTIVE, CARDIAC SHUNT ANALYSIS TECHNIQUE

David L. Gilday, M.D. and
Robert Howman-Giles, M.B.

The Hospital for Sick Children
Toronto, Ontario, Canada

The introduction of the gamma variate function for estimating left to right intracardiac shunts by Maltz and Treves in 1973 (1) began an intense interest in such computer quantification. It rapidly became apparent that certain features were necessary for an ideal shunt detection computer program. These primarily involved the quality of the bolus and the choice of the inflection points. The following is a description of our approximation of this ideal.

METHOD

The radiopharmaceutical must be injected via the external jugular vein to ensure a compact bolus which is essential for adequate quantification. Eleven mCi/square meter body surface of Tc-99m pertechnetate is flushed with 10 cc of saline. The use of a functional image generated from the sequential computer images of the flow through the heart has proved extremely valuable for obtaining the correct placement of the region of interest over the lung. This functional image is the time to peak activity after the bolus has been injected. The regions of interest are easily placed on this functional image to generate time activity histograms. A file on the same disk as the raw data is automatically created to hold the time to peak image (T_{max}), the count maximum for each matrix point image (C_{max}), the regions of interest and the curves. Our current operating system uses a chaining technique so that all pertinent data is carried from the functional image program through all stages to the final analysis.

ANALYSIS

The analysis program initially calculates a bolus score for the transit curve generated for the superior vena cava. This bolus score is equal to the number of seconds required for the activity to rise from 10% of its maximum until it falls to 70% of its maximum. The bolus score should be less than two seconds. If it is greater, then some caution must be observed when reporting the results, as erroneously high shunt values can occur. The data curves are displayed continually during processing. Cursors are automatically positioned on the curve so that the upslope inflection point is equal to 10% of the maximum value and the downslope inflection point is equal to 70% of the maximum on this slope. These cursors may be manuevered via the keyboard to the other appropriate inflection points to obtain a better fit by the least squares fit of the gamma variate function. The fitted curve is displayed on the data curve.

The curves are automatically generated once the regions are established. If the curve is hard to fit due the data then a three-point smooth can be performed at this time and the fitting redone.

For the recirculation curve a special maximum is determined, which is the point which has a significant (10%) drop in counts following it. The recirculation curve is usually much easier to fit if it is smoothed once. The upslope inflection point is that which is closest again to 10% of the maximum, however, the downslope inflection point is the first point after the special maximum. In addition a criterium must be met before the recirculation calculation can be carried out. The first is that the time from 70% inflection point or first transit to the start of shunt recirculation is not too lone, as normal systemic recirculation may intervene.

As the gamma variate fit of each curve is displayed the goodness of fit is calculated. This is the summation of the difference between the raw data and the fitted data squared, divided by the total number of points. This provides numerical confirmation of the visual impression which the operator can then use when assessing the quality of the fitted curve to the raw data. As additional inflection points are chosen, the curve with the best goodness of fit is maintained as a reference curve. When the best curve is finally accepted, this reference curve is used as the gamma variate function fit.

RESULTS

The program has proved to be reliable and also reproducible for different operators. The automatic selection of the first fit inflection points is accepted in nine out of ten cases. Those selected for the recirculation fit are used in three out of five cases. We have found that it is extremely important when studying small children, to double the time interval from .25 seconds to .5 seconds, as the statistics are too low for accurate fitting, which can be done within the analysis program without destroying the original data. In some cases the smoothing is necessary (three-point smooth). Quite frequently the recirculation curve requires a single three-point smooth so as to produce a good curve for the program to fit.

PITFALLS

1. A poor bolus that is strung out will almost always cause a higher result than is found with a compact one.

2. An inadequate number of points on the upslope will not permit the gamma variate function to work.

3. There has to be at least one point after the maximum with a significant drop or the curve will go into outer space.

4. If the data is irregular then a three-point smooth will greatly improve the fitting ability of the gamma variate function.

5. If the counts are low then one of two aids may be employed: a) doubling the time per frame which can be done within the program; or b) using a curve which is generated over both lungs. It must be noted that there can not be any differential flow to lungs which can usually be assessed by looking at the individual lung curves.

6. If the second curve is not smoothed then it is almost always very difficult to get a good fit.

7. A rapid heart rate in a small child may cause a very short normal recirculation time which must not be confused with a shunt.

8. The most difficult single part of this study is the selection of the recirculation special maximum. There is nothing like experience to ensure a good result. However one very helpful hint is to get a good raw data fit that will provide the best possible data for the second fit.

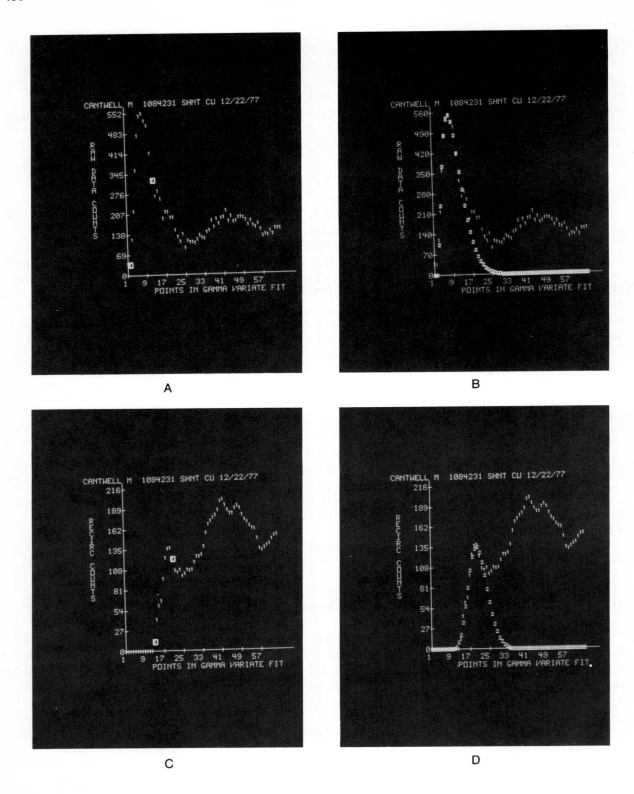

FIG. 1. Curves displayed by the shunt analysis program. (A) Raw data with the computer-selected inflection points. (B) Fit to the raw data, 1 = raw data, 2 = computer fit. (C) Recirculation data with the computer-selected inflection points. (D) Fit to the recirculation, 1 = raw data, 2 = computer fit.

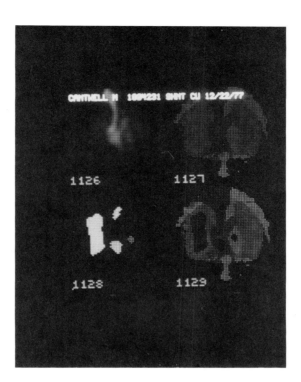

FIG. 2. Display generated by the shunt program of the images and the regions of interest. (Upper left) C_{max} image. (Upper right) T_{max} image. (Lower left) Regions of interest. (Lower right) T_{max} image, regions of interest.

CONCLUSIONS

In 96 childred quantitated by this method resulted in a correlation coefficient of .82 with the dye dilution technique which is considered the most accurate of the catheterization prodedures. A more important statistis is that only six patients were miscategorized. In all these cases the bolus score was not up to par.

REFERENCES

1. Maltz DL, Treves S: Quantitative radionuclide angiocardiography: Determination of Qp : Qs in children. Circulation 47:1049-1056, 1973.

A NEW DIGITAL DISPLAY SYSTEM FOR NUCLEAR VENTRICULOGRAPHY

Charles A. Burnham, John Bradshaw, David Kaufman, Mark Frappier,
Linda A. Deveau, Nathaniel M. Alpert, Gordon L. Brownell

Massachusetts General Hospital
Fruit Street, Boston, MA 02114

ABSTRACT

A scintigraphic display system has been developed which uses
a 64K x 16 Bit MOS memory and standard television monitors. A
64K memory size was chosen to accommodate 32 gated cardiac images.
Its major features include a variable raster size up to 300 x
400 pixels with 1 bit or 8 bits of brightness, a hardware interpolator to allow 64^2 or 128^2 data to be viewed as 256 x 256 x 8
images and independent memories for alphanumeric characters and
cursor.

INTRODUCTION

Applications such as computer assisted nuclear ventriculography have proven the value of digital display techniques. But, they have also indicated the limitations in many existing computer display systems. The situation is now somewhat improved: New general purpose, but relatively low cost, digital display systems have recently been introduced which provide improved image quality (1). In addition, several commercially available scintigraphic data processing systems now provide improved digital image display.

This paper describes a digital display system which was developed at the Massachusetts General Hospital. Its design evolved from a previous interest in display techniques and technology (2,3) as well as a need for a display system suitable for multi-gated nuclear ventriculography.

The availability of fast low-cost memories provides an attractive solution to the problems of storing data accumulated during gated heart studies. When multi-ported, the same memory can also be used as a display buffer. A 128K-byte memory was chosen so as to facilitate a considerable variety of display modes. The display employs a standard EIA 525-line, 60-Hz, interlaced monitor. Its major features are:

1. Hardware to perform linear interperlation between pixels for data raster expansion (X2,X4).
2. Programmable raster size to 300 x 400 pixels of eight or one bit per pixel, (gray scale or graphics).
3. Independent memories for alphanumeric character generator and for cursor position.
4. Minimum need for data formatting.

METHODS

A block diagram of the display is shown in Fig. 1. In order to make effective use of the 128K byte memory for pixel generation a basic pixel period of 132 ns was chosen. As a result image fields with 400 pixels per line and 300 lines may be viewed.

Standard EIA Sync and blanking signals are obtained from a Fairchild 5320 TV sync generator. The Raster Generator uses these signals and four programmable counters to define the raster position and size on the monitor. Clock pulses occurring within the defined raster are counted by a 5th programmed counter and used in addressing the memory. Additional logic modifies the address to provide for interlacing, raster expansion and formatting frames with multiple images.

The pixel generator provides memory requests and formats data for display. It allows for the selection of pixel depth (1 or 8 bits), raster expansion, the cursor and alphanumeric characters. Analog signals are obtained using a commercially available DAC (Hybrid System Model No. 395) and are merged with blanking signals to form an EIA standard composite video signal.

For legability a double sized font (10x14) is used for the alphanumeric characters, which appear as 4 lines of 32 characters per line below the image raster.

A joy stick (Measurement Systems Inc. Model #525) is used in conjunction with the cursor logic and memory, 4K x 1 RAM. The contents of the cursor memory is superimposed as 4K points on a 256 x 256 raster.

The entire display logic has a complexity of about 200 integrated circuits and is implemented on a single 14x14 inch printed circuit board.

Figure 2 depicts the architecture of the system in which the display is incorporated. The external memory was obtained from Electronic Memories and Magnetics Co., Inc. It used 4K static RAM and exhibits a 450-nsec cycle time. The four-port switch includes enable and priority interrupt logic. Control is provided from the computer programmed I/O logic while DMA logic is used to transfer data in block mode. The memory runs interleaved to achieve the data rate necessary for the display.

This architecture ensures simple and straight forward software interactions between the computer and display. The principle preload manipulation is a normalization of data from word format (16-bits) to byte format (8-bits). Display handlers are provided to load the control registers defining the attributes of each displayed frame. Thus picture placement on the screen, raster expansion mode, number of bits per pixel, display of the cursor memory, display of the character memory, and the location of the image in display memory can all be defined.

DISCUSSION

A display system has been developed and incorporated into an existing data processing network (4). It conveniently fulfills a variety of display needs and it has been enthusiastically received by programmers and users. In particular the architecture, large memory, raster expander and graphics capability combine to meet the expanding needs of nuclear medical display systems. The TV format allows monitors, video hard copy units and video recorders to be easily used.

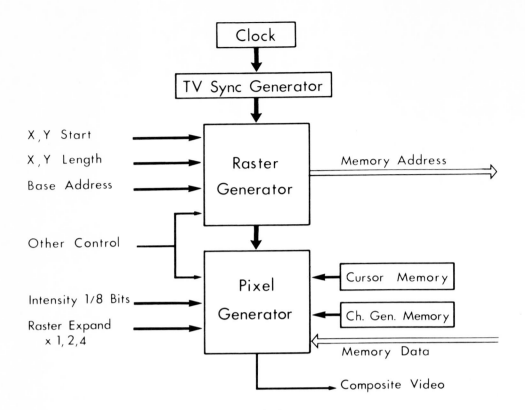

FIG. 1. Display system block diagram.

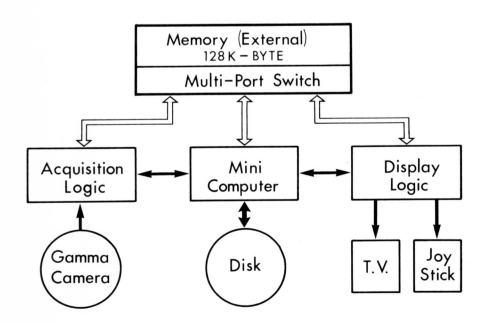

FIG. 2. Data processing system. Block diagram showing relationship of display system with minicomputer and data acquisition.

TABLE 1. TYPICAL DISPLAY MODES

Input Image Matrix	Number Of Images In Memory	Images Per Frame	Raster Expansion	Displayed Raster (1,2,3)
64x64x8	32	1,4,16	x4,x2,x1	256x256x8
128x128x8	8	1,4	x2,x1	256x256x8
256x256x8	2	1	x1	256x256x8
300x400x8 or 1 (4)	1 or 8	1	x1	256x256x8 or 1

(1) Alphanumerics below all displayed images 4 lines of 32 characters may be displayed.

(2) The cursor memory is displayed as 4K points on a 256x256 raster.

(3) Sequential images are timed to multiples of 0.03 sec.

(4) Gray scale or graphics.

REFERENCES

1. Shames, D.M., Farmer, R.E.L., O'Connell, W.: Initial Experience with a High Quality Video Display for Nuclear Medicine Imaging. J. Nucl. Med. 18: 616. June 1977

2. Brownell, G.L., Burnham, C.A., Pizer, S.M., Wilensky, S.: A Computer System for Processing Radioisotope Data from Multiple Sources. Proc. of Symposium on Sharing of Computer Program and Technology in Nuclear Medicine, Oak Ridge, Tenn. April, 1970.

3. Burnham, C.A., Kaufman, D. and Correll, J.E.: A Hardware Interpolator for Display Raster Expansion. Proc. of 3rd. Symposium on Sharing of Computer Programs and Technology in Nuclear Medicine, Miami, FL, June, 1973.

4. Alpert, N.M., Deveau, L.A., Correll, J.E., Burnham, C.A. and Brownell, G.L.: NUMEDICS-II, A distributed resource computer network for nuclear medicine. In Digest of 4th Int. Conf. on Medical Physics, Ottawa, July, 1976

Supported in part by: USPHS Grant #GM16712 - Radioisotope & Data Processing Display

NOTES

NOTES